A COURSEBOOK

on

Language Disorders
in
Children

A COURSEBOOK

on

Language Disorders
in
Children

M. N. Hegde
CALIFORNIA STATE UNIVERSITY-FRESNO

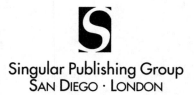

Singular Publishing Group
SAN DIEGO · LONDON

Singular Textbtook Series
Series Editor: M. N. Hegde, Ph.D.

Selected Titles in the Series:
Clinical Methods and Practicum in Speech-Language Pathology by M. N. Hegde, Ph.D., and Deborah Davis, M.A.
Applied Phonetics: The Sounds of American English by Harold T. Edwards, Ph.D.
Applied Phonetics Workbook: A Systematic Approach to Phonetic Transcription by Harold T. Edwards, Ph.D., and Alvin L. Gregg, Ph.D.
The Acoustic Analysis of Speech by Raymond D. Kent, Ph.D., and Charles Read, Ph.D.
Introduction to Sound Acoustics for the Hearing and Speech Sciences by Charles E. Speaks, Ph.D.
Assessement in Speech-Language Pathology: A Resource Manual by Kenneth G. Shipley, Ph.D., and Julie G. McAfee, M.A.
Clinical Speech and Voice Measurement: Laboratory Exercises by Robert F. Orlikoff, Ph.D., and Ronald J. Baken, Ph.D.
Optimizing Theories and Experiments by Randall C. Robey, Ph.D., and Martin C. Schultz. Ph.D.

Also available:
A Singular Manual of Textbook Preparation by M. N. Hegde, Ph.D.

Singular Publishing Group, Inc.
4284 41st Street
San Diego, California 92105-1197

19 Compton Terrace
London, N1 2UN, UK

© 1996 by Singular Publishing Group, Inc.

Printed in the United States of America by McNaughton & Gunn
Typeset in 10/13 Berkeley

Library of Congress Cataloging-in-Publication Data

Hegde, M. N. (Mahabalagiri, N.), 1941–
    A coursebook on language disorders in children / M.N. Hegde.
        p.   cm.
    Includes bibliographical references.
    ISBN 1-56593-618-3
    1. Language disorders in children.   I. Title.
RJ496.L35H44 1995
618.92'855—dc20   95-43670
                                                     CIP

Contents

WRITING A TREATMENT AND MAINTENANCE PLAN
IMPLEMENTING THE TREATMENT PLAN
A NOTE ON COMPREHENSION TRAINING
A NOTE ON THE DEGREE OF STRUCTURE OF TRAINING SESSIONS
REFERENCES AND READING ASSIGNMENTS
STUDY QUESTIONS

Preface

This is a *coursebook* written for courses on children's language disorders, their assessment, and treatment. A coursebook, as described fully under *Introduction*, is both a teaching and a learning tool. I have found the coursebook method of teaching efficient for both the instructor and the student. It is efficient for the instructor because the coursebook provides a lecture outline that he or she can easily expand or modify. It is efficient for the student because it provides important and basic notes already printed.

Many students have given enthusiastic support for the coursebook method of teaching. Also, many instructors across the country who have used my other two coursebooks—one on aphasia and the other on scientific and professional writing—have reinforced the idea that coursebooks are useful teaching and learning tools. I am thankful to all the students and instructors who have given me positive feedback.

This coursebook is written for introductory courses on language disorders in children. It is based on several books including textbooks and journal articles on language disorders in children. The emphasis is on a descriptive and clinical perspective. Attempts have been made to provide extensive information on treatment of language disorders in children. The coursebook makes it easier for instructors to expand the basic information provided here by including complex issues and theoretical perspectives.

Introduction

Effective teaching is a concern of all those who teach. Instructors look for teaching devices that are effective, easy to teach from, and current. They also look for teaching devices that are easily updated. Students, too, look for easy-to-use devices that help them learn without unnecessary effort and frustration. Instructors and students alike look for devices that help integrate lectures and textbook information.

A persistent problem of teaching and learning is that lectures and printed information are not integrated. The two sources of information often are nonparallel, sometimes even contradictory. A frustrating problem for all but a few speed-writing students is accurate note taking in the classroom. But this is mostly an unnecessary problem dictated by the lecture method of instruction and unintegrated printed (textbooks and other sources) and nonprinted (class notes) materials. There should be no need for students to write down in the classroom the definition of terms, outline of topics, major steps of assessment or treatment procedures, arguments, or issues. Such important information should be available in printed form to reduce the pressure of rapid writing.

In spite of their best efforts, the notes most students take are incomplete and may even be inaccurate. Moreover, students who are furiously taking notes on technical and unfamiliar topics cannot listen, understand, reflect, and discuss. When the basic terms, concepts, steps, procedures, summaries, and so forth are given in the form of printed lecture notes, students may find the classroom a more inviting place to discuss, offer comments, and ask questions.

Textbooks, although containing most of the information students need, are not easily integrated with lecture notes. That is why students feel compelled to write down everything an instructor says, including what might be found in their textbooks. Therefore, textbooks do not offer solutions to classroom problems of writing, listening, and discussing. A coursebook is designed to solve these classroom problems students face. It is a teaching tool that helps both the student and the instructor.

WHAT IS A COURSEBOOK?

A coursebook is an unusual teaching tool that offers printed class notes on the left-half of each page and empty space on the right-half to take additional notes. It is a multipurpose book.

A *coursebook* does:

- give printed notes and room for taking lecture notes

- give important terms and defines them for the student

- list major points of arguments and issues

- give basic information in the form of tables and summaries

- list steps, procedures, methods, techniques and their advantages and limitations

- reduce the pressure of note taking

- provide a single source of integrated information collected from multiple sources

A *coursebook* does not:

- present detailed arguments and issues

- present research and data in detail

- give in-depth reviews of controversies

- give detailed description of theories

- explore research bases of theories in detail

- examine future trends

- suggest research needs

Therefore:

- **A coursebook does not replace a textbook**

A coursebook is a companion to one or more textbooks. Students should carefully study their textbooks and then use this coursebook to get summarized information integrated with information offered in the class and obtained from journals and other, more recent sources.

A textbook is written for the student. A coursebook is written both for the student and the instructor. For the instructor, a coursebook lightens the load of course preparation and for the student, it lightens the load of taking accurate class notes. For both the student and the instructor, it serves many common purposes because it is both a learning and a teaching tool.

WHAT THIS BOOK DOES FOR THE STUDENT

- The left-half of each page offers summarized information from multiple sources.

- The student can think of this book as basic class notes already printed for his or her convenience. Therefore, the student does not need to write as much while listening to the lectures. All technical terms, definitions, and major points that most instructors are likely to offer in a class are already printed for the student.

- The printed information has been gathered from multiple sources, including journal articles and leading textbooks. Thus, it offers information collected from multiple sources, much like what an instructor does in teaching a course.

- The right-half of all pages are empty so that students can write notes on them. Students need to write only new information, additional examples, and expansions that the instructor offers in the class. The hand-written notes are more likely to be unique and newer information and perspectives the individual instructors offer.

- The empty portions of each page also may be used out of classrooms. For instance, the student can take notes from journal articles or newer books read at home or at the library.

- When used properly, a coursebook makes a single, integrated, updated source of information on a topic.

- Properly completed and updated coursebooks can be a valuable reference for clinical work and for studying for master's degree comprehensive examinations and the national examination for ASHA certification.

WHAT THIS BOOK DOES FOR THE INSTRUCTOR

- Foremost, a coursebook is an instructional package already prepared for the instructor.

- The instructor may use the printed information as lecture notes and outlines.

- Therefore, this book saves much time and effort preparing for the class.

- The information is gathered from several books, although the information is based on a few leading texts.

- The book provides selected information printed such that it may be directly copied on transparencies for overhead projection.

- On the blank right-hand side of each page, the instructor may write additional notes, examples, reminders, and other devices used during the lecture. Recent research studies published in journals, references, and so forth also may be written on the right-hand side. The empty space may also be used to write down student assignments. In essence, both the instructor and the student will use the blank portions of pages in much the same way: to write additional information.

- The book reduces the need to repeat or dictate information, especially technical terms and their definitions. Instructors know that much classroom time is wasted in this unnecessary activity.

- The book may help instructors reduce the unwanted variability in student note taking.

Once again, this coursebook does not stand alone. It should be used along with a textbook of the instructor's choice.

Note: Most of this standard introduction to coursebooks is reprinted from Hegde, M. N. (1994): *A coursebook on aphasia and other neurogenic language disorders*. San Diego: Singular Publishing Group. Reprinted with permission.

UNIT 1

An Overview of Language

. . . .

- Speech and Language

- The Linguistic Analysis of Language

- The Behavioral Analysis of Language

- Nonverbal Communication

- Comprehension and Production

- Language and Culture

- References and Reading Assignments

- Study Questions

. . . .

SPEECH AND LANGUAGE

Language can be verbal or nonverbal.

Language is broader than speech; you cannot produce oral language without speech. However, you can produce non-oral language without speech.

You can produce speech without language because speech is a smaller building block of the larger behavioral unit called language.

Language has typically been defined by linguists or psycholinguists as a mental system of arbitrarily selected codes that represent ideas about the world.

Members of a verbal community conventionally agree upon codes; that is why they are arbitrary.

Speech is the actual production of language.

THE LINGUISTIC ANALYSIS OF LANGUAGE

Linguistic analysis typically is concerned with the **structure** of language. These structures may be described as **components** of language.

The following are the linguistic components of language:

- phonologic component

- semantic component

- syntactic component

- morphologic component

- pragmatic component

Each of these components, except for the syntactic, has a study associated with it: phonology, semantics, morphology, and pragmatics.

UNIT NOTES

CLASS NOTES

Phonology is the study of the sound system of languages and the rules of combining phonemes to form meaningful words.

The phonologic component is an aspect of language; it is the production of speech sounds and the organization of sounds according to certain rules.

Phonemes are basic sound elements that can make a difference in meaning.

Semantics is the study of meaning in language.

Semanticists are those who specialize in the study of meaning.

The **semantic component** of language is the element of meaning in language.

There are different kinds of meaning.

Referential meaning. Meaning conveyed by words that refer to things and objects.

Connotative meaning. Emotionally associated meaning suggested by words.

Relational meaning. Meaning conveyed by words that are related to each other in some sense.

Most words have multiple meanings.

Syntax is a collection of rules about word combinations and sentence forms.

Syntax is a part of **grammar**; besides syntax, grammar includes the morphologic component of language.

Remember that grammar is a broader term that includes morphology and syntax.

Morphology is the study of word structures. As already noted, it is a part of grammar.

Morphology is concerned with the small elements of grammar including grammatic morphemes (the regular plural and the possessive inflection, the present progressive *ing*, the auxiliary and copula, articles, prepositions, conjunctions, pronouns, the regular past tense inflection, the irregular plural and the past are examples of grammatic morphemes of English).

Morphemes are the smallest meaningful units of language.

Morphemes are classified either as roots and affixes or as free and bound.

Roots: Words that cannot be divided.

Affixes: Morphemes that are added to roots. There are two kinds of affixes:

    Prefixes: Morphemes that are attached at the beginning of roots (*re* in *redo* and *un* in *undo*)

    Suffixes: Morphemes that are attached at the end of roots (*s* in *books* and *ing* in *walking*)

Free morphemes: They can stand alone and convey meaning (most words).

Bound morphemes: They are combined with other morphemes; cannot stand alone (the plural *s* or the present progressive *ing*).

Pragmatics is the study of language use in social contexts. It specifies the rules of language usage.

Pragmatics places greater emphasis on the functional (usage) aspect of language. It is concerned with pragmatic communication skills which include:

• Maintaining eye contact during communication

• Initiating conversation

• Taking turns in a conversational exchange

• Maintaining conversation on a given topic

• Time-, situation-, and topic-appropriate speech

• Narrative skills

THE BEHAVIORAL ANALYSIS OF LANGUAGE

The behavioral analysis of language is more concerned with the functional units of verbal behaviors than with the structural units or components.

Skinner, whose behavioral analysis holds much clinical relevance, suggests that *verbal behavior* is a better term than *language*.

While the term *language* often means a mental or linguistic system, the term *verbal behavior* means actions.

Skinner defined **verbal behavior** as a class of social behavior shaped and maintained by the members of a verbal community.

Skinner analyzed verbal behaviors in terms of such functional units as mands, tacts, echoics, intraverbals, and autoclitics.

In the behavioral analysis, a **functional unit** is a cause-effect relation. Note that the term *functional* in the behavioral analysis does not suggest use as it normally does.

Instead of looking at the structure of verbal responses (as linguists do), Skinner looked at the causes and effects of verbal responses.

All verbal responses that have the same or similar causes and consequences and produce similar effects on the listener are grouped together as a **functional unit**.

A functional unit may be a word, a phrase, or a sentence or an extended utterance.

Mands are verbal responses that have motivational states as causes and they are influenced by primary (unconditioned) reinforcers.

Mands include all requests, commands, demands, and similar expressions.

A **tact** is a group of verbal responses whose cause is a state of affairs in the environment; reinforcers are social. A tact often is a descriptive statement. Environmental events and objects are the stimuli for tacts.

An **echoic** is an imitated response; the cause is another speaker's verbal response (the modeled stimulus).

Intraverbals are verbal responses whose cause or causes are the speaker's own prior verbal responses. A speaker's prior speech is stimuli for subsequent speech (intraverbals). When something you said is stimulus for you to say more, we have intraverbals.

Most proverbs, alphabets, counting, and so forth are examples of intraverbals.

Much of fluent speech is due to intraverbals because one word or phrase causes you to say more.

Autoclitics include the traditional elements of grammar.

Autoclitics often describe some aspect of the causes of other verbal behaviors.

For example, when you use a plural inflection /s/ in a sentence like "I see two cups," you are in effect specifying the quantitative aspect of the events that caused your statement. Or, when you say that *I see in the newspaper that* it is going to rain tomorrow," one part of the statement (italicized) explains why you are saying that it is going to rain tomorrow. The italicized portion is an autoclitic.

As you will find out later, the principles of behavior change are frequently used in the treatment of language disorders.

NONVERBAL COMMUNICATION

Communication may be verbal or nonverbal; language also may be verbal or nonverbal.

UNIT NOTES

Nonverbal languages are not spoken. They use signs, gestures, and nonvocal symbols.

American Sign Language is a prime example of a nonverbal language or system of communication.

Systems that include symbols to communicate include **Blissymbolics** and the **Carrier symbols**.

The **rebus system** uses pictures to communicate.

COMPREHENSION AND PRODUCTION

The terms **comprehension** and **receptive language** are used to suggest the process of attending to and understanding expressed language (verbal or nonverbal).

The actual speaking of a language is called **production**.

Generally, comprehension of language precedes production.

However, children can produce structures they do not comprehend.

LANGUAGE AND CULTURE

Language and culture are closely related. Language is a vehicle for cultural transmission.

Acquisition, production, and use of language are a cultural phenomenon.

To appropriately diagnose and treat language disorders, the clinician needs to understand the cultural background of the client. We will find out more about this in Unit 8.

Instructor's Views and Critical Comments on the Components and the Study of Language

_____

_____

_____

_____

_____

_____

_____

_____

_____

_____

_____

_____

_____

_____

_____

_____

_____

_____

_____

_____

_____

REFERENCES AND READING ASSIGNMENTS

Nelson, N. W. (1993). *Childhood language disorders in context.* New York: Macmillan

Read Chapter 2 for an overview of language and its components.

Reed, V. (1994). *An introduction to children with language disorders.* New York: Macmillan.

Read Chapter 1 for an overview of language and its components.

For a more detailed study of language and language acquisition, consult the following textbooks. Review your notes from your course on language acquisition (or development):

Gleason, J. B. (1993). *The development of language* (3rd. ed.). New York: Macmillan.

Owens, R. E. (1992). *Language development: An introduction* (3rd. ed.). New York: Macmillan.

Special Assignments From the Instructor:

_____

_____

_____

_____

_____

_____

_____

_____

_____

_____

_____

_____

_____

_____

_____

_____

_____

_____

_____

_____

_____

_____

_____

_____

_____

STUDY QUESTIONS

1. What is speech?

   _____

   _____

   _____

2. What is language?

   _____

   _____

   _____

   _____

3. List the five components of language:

   I. _____   II. _____

   III. _____   IV. _____

   V. _____

4. Define phonology:

   _____

   _____

   _____

5. Define semantics:

   _____

   _____

6. Distinguish between referential and connotative meanings:

   _____

   _____

   _____

7. What is syntax?

   _____

   _____

8. Define morphology:

9. Define the following terms:

Grammatic morphemes

Bound morphemes

Free morphemes

Prefixes and suffixes

10. What is pragmatics?

11. What is Skinner's word for language? _____

12. Define a functional unit:

13. What are mands?

14. What are tacts?

15. What are intraverbals?

_____

_____

16. What is Skinner's term for grammar?_____

17. What is an echoic?

_____

_____

18. Define nonverbal communication:

_____

_____

19. Distinguish between comprehension and production:

_____

_____

_____

20. Is comprehension always ahead of production?

_____

UNIT 2

An Overview of Language Disorders in Children

. . . .

- Prevalence of Language Disorders

- Effects of Language Disorders

- What is a Language Disorder?

- A Basic Description of Language Disorders

- Classification of Language Disorders

- Explanation of Language Disorders

- References and Reading Assignments

- Study Questions

. . . .

PREVALENCE OF LANGUAGE DISORDERS

Precise and reliable information on the prevalence of language disorders in children is not available. Literature suggests that:

- The numbers vary across age groups.

- Some children with language disorders may be diagnosed as learning disabled and hence not counted.

- Some children are late bloomers.

- Ten to 15% of 2-year-olds, and 4 to 7.5% of 3-year-olds may show some degree of language delay.

- An unspecified number of children may show subtle language problems that are not easily detected.

- Even some or most of the late bloomers may have undetected residual problems.

- More boys than girls show language impairment (ratios range from 3:1 to 15:1).

See Reed (1994) for a complete discussion of issues.

EFFECTS OF LANGUAGE DISORDERS

Language problems of childhood have far reaching consequences. Language problems affect the child's social behavior and educational achievement. Many children with learning disabilities have language impairment. Language disorders that persist into adulthood can cause serious occupational difficulties.

Because of such serious consequences, assessment and treatment of language disorders is an important part of the duties of the speech-language pathologist.

UNIT NOTES

CLASS NOTES

The speech-language pathologist's involvement with language is somewhat recent. The 1960s witnessed the growth of information on language development and disorders in children. Speech-language pathologists were influenced by:

- various theories of language, especially those of the linguists and psycholinguists

- the behavioral methods of treating language disorders

Currently, the speech-language pathologist is greatly involved in the study and treatment of language and its disorders in all age groups.

This coursebook is concerned with the language disorders of children.

WHAT IS A LANGUAGE DISORDER?

There is no single definition of language disorder that most experts accept. The term applies to a heterogeneous group of children who show diverse problems in the acquisition, comprehension, production, and use of various aspects of language.

Some children who exhibit language disorders have associated conditions such as mental retardation and hearing impairment. Many other children who exhibit language disorders do not exhibit other serious problems: a language disorder is their only significant problem.

Each group exhibits some unique behaviors that are usually attributed to the associated condition; but all groups share many common characteristics of language problems.

The following terms are found in the literature, but experts do not agree on their precise definitions:

Language disorder: There are at least three views on what language disorder is:

- *Normative View of Language Disorders*
  Language performance below what is expected based either on mental age, chronological age, or specific measures of language.

- *Pathological View of Language Disorders*
  A pattern of deficient language that is abnormal, deviant, unusual (not found in children who speak normally).

- *Pragmatic View of Language Disorders*
  Language skills that do not help meet the social and educational demands made on the child.

Some but not all clinicians believe that the term *language disorders* necessarily implies an unusual, abnormal process. It is not the same as delayed language; disordered language is not the language of a younger child; it is abnormal. Disordered language is acquired at a different rate and in unusual sequences. The skills acquired may be different from those acquired by children who are developing normally. Children with language disorders may exhibit uneven abilities across different aspects of language; the children's vocabulary may be large enough to support syntax, but there may be no syntactic structures, for example.

- **Language delay:** This means that the child is learning language at a slower than normal rate; but the sequence is normal and the skills acquired are not bizarre. The term may suggest that the child with language delay will catch up with the normal rate, but data do not suggest this. Some do catch up and some do not and some of those who do may retain subtle deficits. Typically, there is no implication that the observed pattern of language is abnormal, deviant, bizarre, or unusual. An older child simply shows the language skills of a younger child, and may or may not continue to show deficiencies.

- **Language impairment:** Often includes the same meanings as the term *language disorder*.

- **Language deficiency:** The meaning is perhaps closer to that of *language delay*.

- **Language problems**: A more general term that may imply a delay or disorder.

- **Language handicap**: A more general term that tends to emphasize the negative effects of the disorder or delay.

A BASIC DESCRIPTION OF LANGUAGE DISORDERS

If we look at the **language problems that are common to this heterogeneous group of children**, we may describe language disorders as:

- **Limited amount of language:** Children with language problems almost always show a deficiency in the quantity of language learned, comprehended, and produced. These children have a limited verbal repertoire.

- **Deficient grammar:** Children with language disorders typically have difficulty in learning, comprehending, and producing aspects of grammar. The children's speech shows gross or subtle deficiencies in morphologic as well as syntactic aspects.

- **Deficient or inappropriate use:** Children with language disorders are less proficient in using whatever the amount of language that has been mastered; often, the child's use of language may not be appropriate to the time, place, person, and topic of conversation. Other pragmatic problems (to be described later) also characterize language problems.

A description of language disorders, such as the one just given, is not etiological, and is only a shorthand description of the basic problems of children with language disorders.

Throughout this book, while recognizing the differences of opinion, the various terms are used interchangeably. As used in this book, the terms:

UNIT NOTES

- *Language delay* does not necessarily suggest that the children showing it will overcome it.

- *Language disorder* does not necessarily mean that the process or the product is abnormal or bizarre.

Please remember this as you read this book. Also remember that some experts use terms with certain exclusive meanings.

CLASSIFICATION OF LANGUAGE DISORDERS

Experts disagree on classifying language disorders. Among the different classifications, the following are common:

Etiological Classification: Classification based on presumed or demonstrated etiology of the disorder. This is influenced by the medical model.

The problem here is that in many cases, causes of language disorders cannot be found.

Even when a language problem is associated with an obvious condition such as mental retardation or autism, it is not possible to conclude that one is the cause of the other. The retardation and the language disorder are both aspects of one problem; there is no justification to assume that retardation is the cause and the language difficulty is the effect.

Descriptive Classification: This classification avoids the etiological approach because of the difficulty in finding causes. The main task is to describe the language characteristics of children who have problems.

The problem with this classification is that causes are important. We need to look for them. Causes explain effects and in some cases, may lead to more effective treatment.

Nonetheless, it is important to recognize that in many cases, the **original** or **instigating** causes are difficult to determine.

We may have better opportunities to find out the **maintaining causes.**

EXPLANATION OF LANGUAGE DISORDERS

Explanations describe causes of events or effects we try to understand.

There are various explanations. None are totally satisfactory to all or even most of the experts; each has serious limitations.

Explanation Based on Concomitant Pathology

Language disorders are caused by associated clinical or pathological conditions.

For instance, language disorders are caused by such concomitant clinical conditions as developmental disabilities (including mental retardation and autism), hearing loss, traumatic brain injury early in infancy, or emotional and behavioral disorders. Language disabilities and such clinical conditions often are associated.

The problem with this explanation is that language disorders and each of the concomitant clinical conditions are a part of the single problem. One part of a problem does not explain the other parts. Does mental retardation explain language disorders or do both need an explanation?

Explanation Based on Underlying Deficits

Language disorders are due to deficits in certain functions, abilities, or processes that presumably underlie language skills.

For instance, language disorders may be due to deficits in cognitive or perceptual functions including auditory and visual perception and processing, tactile discrimination, spatial memory, motor skills including speed and coordination, abstraction, cross-modal integration, and so forth.

One problem with this explanation is that language deficits themselves may be responsible for some or most of the cognitive deficits. Did the language problem come first or the cognitive deficits? Causes come first, effects later. Another problem is that treating the underlying deficit or the cause (cognitive deficiencies) should result in improved language. This does not necessarily happen.

Explanation Based on Normal Variation

This is an explanation that applies particularly to a group of children who show language disorders but no gross pathology or concomitant clinical condition that can explain the disorder.

Language disorders in such children are called specific language impairment, described in Unit 3.

Language disorders are not pathologically based, but are a reflection of the normal variation in linguistic skills.

Just as some people are deficient in musical skills or spatial skills, some children are deficient in language skills. Language skills are like other social and intellectual skills that vary across children. Those at the lower end of the normal variation may seem to have a disorder, but there is no disorder because they just have limited skills (Leonard, 1991; Dale & Cole, 1991).

The normal variation explanation is especially applicable to **specific language impairment**. The advocates of this explanation recognize that in some children, language disorder is associated with disease or injury to the nervous system. Therefore, the explanation only says that pathological conditions are not always necessary bases for limited language skills.

Critics of the normal variation viewpoint out that some children exhibit such serious problems in learning language that some pathological factors or deficiency in underlying processes must be involved.

Multiple Conditions and Causes

Children with language disorders are a heterogeneous group. Therefore, the causes also are multiple, and varied across children.

Most experts believe that language disorders have multiple causes. Different subgroups may have different sets of multiple causes. In the subsequent units, we will consider various associated conditions and potential causes of language disorders. These include genetic, neurophysiological, sensory, and environmental factors.

Instructor's Views and Critical Comments on Explaining Language Disorders _____

_____

_____

_____

_____

_____

_____

_____

_____

_____

_____

_____

_____

_____

_____

_____

_____

_____

_____

_____

_____

_____

_____

REFERENCES AND READING ASSIGNMENTS

Dale, P. S., & Cole, K. N. (1991). What's normal? Specific language impairment in an individual difference perspective. *Language, Speech, and Hearing Services in Schools, 22*(2), 80–83.

Read this article to understand the view that language disorders suggest individual differences in language skills.

Johnston, J. R. (1991). The continuing relevance of cause: A reply to Leonard's "Specific language impairment as a clinical category." *Language, Speech, and Hearing Services in Schools, 22*(2), 75–79.

Read this article to understand the view that language disorders may be due to underlying deficits.

Leonard, L. B. (1991). Specific language impairment as a clinical category. *Language, Speech, and Hearing Services in Schools, 22*(2), 66–68.

Read this paper to understand the view that language disorders may reflect normal variation in language skills.

Nelson, N. W. (1993). *Childhood language disorders in context.* New York: Macmillan.

Read Chapter 4 for a discussion of definitions and potential causes of language disorders.

Paul, R. (1995). *Language disorders from infancy through adolescence: Assessment and intervention.* St. Louis: Mosby.

Read Chapter 1 for a discussion of definition and models of language disorders.

Reed, V. (1994). *An introduction to children with language disorders.* New York: Macmillan.

Read Chapter 4 for an overview of language disorders.

Special Assignments From the Instructor:

_____

_____

_____

_____

_____

_____

_____

_____

_____

_____

_____

_____

_____

_____

_____

_____

_____

_____

_____

_____

_____

STUDY QUESTIONS

1. Summarize the information on the prevalence of language disorders in children:

   _____

   _____

   _____

   _____

2. What are some of the far-reaching consequences of language disorders in children?

   _____

   _____

   _____

   _____

3. What was the most significant impact of the behavioral approach?

   _____

   _____

   _____

   _____

4. How did linguistics influence speech-language pathologists?

   _____

   _____

   _____

   _____

5. Describe the three kinds of problems that are common to most if not all children who exhibit language disorders:

   _____

   _____

   _____

   _____

_____

_____

6. Define the following terms:

Language disorders

_____

_____

_____

_____

Language delay

_____

_____

_____

_____

Specific language impairment

_____

_____

_____

_____

_____

7. Distinguish between etiological and descriptive classification of language disorders:

_____

_____

_____

_____

8. What is an instigating or original cause of language disorder?

_____

_____

9. How would you demonstrate that a certain cause has been maintaining a language disorder?

_____

_____

_____

_____

_____

10. What is an explanation of language disorders based on concomitant pathological conditions?

_____

_____

_____

_____

_____

11. What is an explanation based on underlying deficits?

_____

_____

_____

_____

_____

12. What is an explanation based on normal variation?

_____

_____

_____

_____

_____

UNIT 3

Specific Language Impairment

. . . .

- Risk Factors for Language Disorders in Children

- Language Characteristics of Children with SLI

- Is SLI Truly Specific to Language?

- Explanation of SLI

- Treatment of Specific Language Impairment

- References and Reading Assignments

- Study Questions

. . . .

Some children who exhibit a language disorder may have associated clinical conditions. For example, some children with language disorders have associated mental retardation, brain injury, hearing impairment, and autism. Their language disorder is a part of a larger clinical picture.

Many children who exhibit a language disorder, however, do not have any serious concomitant problems. They appear normal except for their language problem. They may have deficiencies in certain cognitive functions, but associated problems, if discovered, do not explain the language disorder. The language disorder in such children is called **specific language impairment (SLI)**, which is essentially language impairment with no known associated, explanatory clinical condition. The term suggests that the impairment is specific to language and no other impairment of significance or relevance is found in such children.

Language problems that are now diagnosed as SLI were often diagnosed as **congenital** or **childhood aphasia** in the past. Like specific language impairment, congenital aphasia is language disorder in children who are otherwise normal. Brain injury or dysfunction was hypothesized but never satisfactorily demonstrated.

Sometimes, SLI in infants and toddlers is described as **slow expressive language development (SELD)**.

RISK FACTORS FOR LANGUAGE DISORDERS IN INFANTS

The following risk factors observed during infancy suggest that the child may later have language disorders whether diagnosed as SLI, SELD, or some other category:

- serious prematurity with very low birth weight

- presence of various genetic syndromes

- maternal drug abuse including alcoholism

- any natal condition that causes brain injury

- sensory deficits, especially hearing impairment

- physical disabilities and frequent illness resulting in prolonged hospitalization

- neglect and abuse

- delayed babbling

- lack of eye contact (mutual gaze)

- lack of joint attention

- lack of smiling

- lack of play activities

- reduced use of gestures

- early phonological difficulties

LANGUAGE CHARACTERISTICS OF CHILDREN WITH SLI

- The sequence of language acquisition is generally the same as that for children who are normally developing

- An asynchronous profile of language development may be evident as in children with Down syndrome (different degrees of deficiency in different aspects of language)

- Generally better pragmatic skills than syntactic and morphological skills are demonstrated (unlike children with autism)

The characteristics of SLI in toddlers and preschoolers include deficiencies in prelinguistic behaviors and phonologic, semantic, morphologic, syntactic, and pragmatic problems.

Prelinguistic Behavioral Deficiencies

- Difficulty in establishing mutual gaze, eye contact

- Difficulty in exhibiting mutual attention with an adult (following an adult's lead in paying attention to objects and events)

- Greater use of gestures and vocalizations than words and phrases to communicate needs

- Less complex babbling with fewer consonants

Phonological Problems

- Articulatory and phonologic problems frequently are found in children with SLI

- Poor intelligibility of speech

- Possibility of improved intelligibility by school age

- Phonological problems are a potential indicator of later language problems

- Consonants not yet produced retard the acquisition of words starting with those consonants

Semantic Problems

- Delay in learning the first few words

- Slow rate of word acquisition, especially between 18 and 24 months when normally there is a sudden spurt in learning words

- Both overly generalized and overly restricted use of words

- Use of general, instead of specific words (e.g., the use of *this*, and *that*, instead of particular words)

- Difficulty in using words they understand

• Word finding problems which result in dysfluencies including pauses (hesitations), interjections (*fillers*), and repetitions

Morphologic Problems

Morphologic problems are especially marked in children with SLI. These problems include omissions of:

• regular and irregular plural morphemes

• possessive morphemes

• present progressive

• third person singular

• articles

• auxiliary and copula verbs

• regular and irregular past tense inflections

Besides omission, children with SLI may show confusion between:

• the singular and plural forms of words

• the plural and singular forms of auxiliary and copula (*are/is*)

• subject case markings (*him* for *he* or *her* for *she*)

• regular and irregular forms of plural and past tense morphemes

Multiple **explanations** have been offered to account for morphologic problems in children with SLI:

Perceptual explanation: Children **do not perceive morphologic features** as well as the other words; omitted morphologic features are not salient in the speech they hear (produced with low intensity, less stress).

Syntactic explanation: Difficulties are due not so much to perceptual difficulties, but to syntactic complexities.

Semantic explanation: The morphologic difficulties are due to semantic redundancy of morphological features in speech (not critical for meaning).

All three factors, along with other unrecognized factors, may be involved.

Syntactic Problems

• Shorter utterances

• Few transformations (limited sentence types)

• Slow increase in sentence complexity

• Slow increase in sentence variety

Pragmatic Problems

• Reluctance to initiate conversation or initiation at inappropriate times

• Fewer comments on events and persons

• Difficulty in describing events, pictures, and other stimuli

• Interactions often limited to answering questions asked

• Fewer **joint attentional interactions** (e.g., the child and the mother looking at the same object and talking about it or manipulating it)

• Limited use of gestures

• Passivity in conversational interactions

• Inappropriate turn taking

UNIT NOTES

- Difficulty in sustaining topic of conversation

- Irrelevant comments

- Deficient **conversational repair strategies** (e.g., difficulty in asking for clarification when messages are not understood)

- Deficient narrative skills (repetition, lack of new information, lack of chronological sequence)

- Greater difficulty in interacting with peers (e.g., children with SLI may be more willing to talk to adults than to their peers)

IS SLI TRULY SPECIFIC TO LANGUAGE?

Some experts think not. Note that the concept of specific language impairment is based on the idea that the children have no other problems of significance or relevance. However, when it is suggested that they have related problems, then the diagnostic category is essentially questioned.

Research has suggested problems in cognitive skills and sensory functions in some of the children with SLI:

- Attentional deficits

- Tendency toward hyperactivity

- Difficulty interpreting rapidly sequenced auditory or visual stimuli

- Difficulty with complex reasoning tasks

- Difficulty with symbolic play activities

- Problems in haptic (touch) perception

- Problems with object classification

Note that not all children with SLI have shown such deficiencies. Some children do seem to have difficulties limited to language functions.

Prognosis

Toddlers and preschoolers with SLI are likely to be diagnosed as **learning disabled** in grade school. Thus the children with SLI are likely to experience academic problems.

Those with improved expressive language may still have difficulty with advanced, complex, or subtle language skills.

Children with SLI are likely to show deficient socialization in school even when their expressive language skills improve significantly.

Children with SLI who also have general behavior problems tend to do worse than those without such problems.

EXPLANATION OF SLI

Explanations of SLI share certain concepts used in explaining language disorders in general (See Unit 2: *An overview of language disorders in children*).

There are two major explanations of SLI: Explanation based on underlying deficits and that based on normal variation.

Explanation Based on Underlying Deficits

SLI is due to deficits that underlie language functions. In children with SLI, cognitive, auditory, perceptual, intellectual, and other factors that underlie language may be abnormal.

As noted earlier, children with specific language impairment have difficulty in interpreting any rapidly presented sequenced events (auditory or visual) and in working on complex reasoning tasks. Such difficulties may be the underlying deficits of SLI (Johnston, 1991).

Explanation Based on Normal Variation

Specific language impairment is not pathologically based, but is a reflection of the normal variation in linguistic skills. Just as some people are deficient in musical skills or spatial skills, some children are deficient in language skills.

Language skills are like other social and intellectual skills that vary across children. Those at the lower end of the normal variation may seem to have a disorder, but there is no disorder because they just have limited skills (Leonard, 1991; Dale & Cole, 1991).

The advocates of normal variation in language skills as an explanation of SLI recognize that in some children, language disorder is associated with disease or injury to the nervous system. The advocates also recognize that in many children, language disorders may be associated with other clinical conditions (e.g., mental retardation or hearing impairment). Therefore, the explanation only says that pathological conditions are not always necessary bases for limited language skills.

TREATMENT OF SPECIFIC LANGUAGE IMPAIRMENT

See Units 10 through 13 for treatment procedures of language disorders, procedural variations, and maintenance procedures.

Instructor's Views and Critical Comments on Specific Language Disorders in Children _____

_____

_____

_____

_____

_____

_____

_____

_____

_____

_____

_____

_____

_____

_____

_____

_____

_____

_____

_____

_____

_____

REFERENCES AND READING ASSIGNMENTS

Dale, P. S., & Cole, K. N. (1991). What's normal? Specific language impairment in an individual difference perspective. *Language, Speech, and Hearing Services in Schools,* 22(2), 80–83.

Read this article to understand the view that language disorders suggest individual differences in language skills, not necessarily pathological conditions.

Johnston, J. R. (1991). The continuing relevance of cause: A reply to Leonard's "Specific language impairment as a clinical category." *Language, Speech, and Hearing Services in Schools,* 22(2), 75–79.

Read this article for a defense of the view that specific language impairment is a clinical category.

Leonard, L. B. (1991). Specific language impairment as a clinical category. *Language, Speech, and Hearing Services in Schools,* 22(2), 66–68.

Read this paper to understand the objections to the concept of specific language impairment and the view that language disorders may be better viewed as limited language skills with no implication of pathology.

Nelson, N. W. (1993). *Childhood language disorders in context.* New York: Macmillan.

Read Chapter 4 for a discussion of definitions and potential causes of language disorders.

Paul, R. (1995). *Language disorders from infancy through adolescence: Assessment and intervention.* St. Louis: Mosby.

Read Chapter 1 for a discussion of definition and models of language disorders.

Reed, V. (1994). *An introduction to children with language disorders.* New York: Macmillan.

Read Chapter 4 for an overview of language disorders.

Special Assignments From the Instructor:

_____

_____

_____

_____

_____

_____

_____

_____

_____

_____

_____

_____

_____

_____

_____

_____

_____

_____

_____

_____

_____

STUDY QUESTIONS

1. Define specific language impairment (SLI):

   _____

   _____

   _____

   _____

2. What was an earlier name for specific language impairment?

   _____

3. In whom is the slow expressive language development (SELD) diagnosed?

   _____

4. List at least 10 risk factors for language disorders that may be observed in infants:

   1. _____   2. _____

   3. _____   4. _____

   5. _____   6. _____

   7. _____   8. _____

   9. _____   10. _____

5. Do children with SLI generally follow the normal sequence of language acquisition?:

   _____

6. What is asynchronous language development?

   _____

   _____

   _____

   _____

7. Describe the prelinguistic behavioral deficiencies of children with SLI:

   _____

   _____

   _____

_____

_____

8. Summarize the semantic problems experienced by children with SLI:

_____

_____

_____

_____

_____

9. Summarize the morphologic problems experienced by children with SLI.

_____

_____

_____

_____

_____

10. What is a perceptual explanation of morphological problems experienced by children with SLI?

_____

_____

_____

_____

_____

11. Summarize the pragmatic problems experienced by children with SLI:

_____

_____

_____

_____

_____

12. How do you answer the question "Is SLI truly specific to language?"

_____

_____

_____

_____

_____

13. State the explanation of SLI based on underlying deficits:

_____

_____

_____

_____

_____

_____

_____

14. State the explanation of SLI based on normal variation:

_____

_____

_____

_____

_____

15. Compare and contrast the two explanations of SLI. Which one do you prefer and why?

_____

_____

_____

_____

_____

_____

UNIT 4

Mental Retardation and Language Disorders

Language disorders are a common characteristic of mental retardation. Many children treated for language disorders in speech and hearing clinics have various degrees of mental retardation. A basic understanding of mental retardation, including its common causes or associated conditions, is essential to design and implement language treatment programs for these children. Therefore, in this unit you will study mental retardation, its potential causes, and associated language disorders.

DEFINITION OF MENTAL RETARDATION

The American Association on Mental Deficiency defines mental retardation as "significantly subaverage general intellectual functioning existing concurrently with deficits in adaptive behavior, and manifested during the developmental period" (Grossman, 1983, p. 1). The developmental period extends up to age 18.

Individuals who are mentally retarded show deficits in almost all aspects of life. Many individuals who are profoundly retarded are institutionalized because they need constant supervision and care. Others who are less retarded may hold a job and raise a family. There are many individuals between these two extremes who need special services to various extents. In the schools, the children who are retarded often are found in special educational programs.

SOME PRESUMED OR DEMONSTRATED CAUSES OF MENTAL RETARDATION

Mental retardation has many causes. Most of these causes are presumed because of their frequent association with retardation. Some of the causes are environmentally induced whereas others are genetic (inherited). However, even genetic causes may have an environmental origin. Certain poisonous chemicals may induce genetic mutations or abnormalities which cause retardation in the offspring.

The factors that are associated with mental retardation are classified in different ways. No classification is exhaustive, as new conditions that are associated with retardation emerge periodically. The following is but one method of classification:

- Mental retardation associated with prenatal infections or toxicity

- Mental retardation associated with natal conditions

- Mental retardation associated with postnatal poisonings or toxicity

- Mental retardation associated with head trauma

- Mental retardation associated with metabolic disorders

- Mental retardation associated with endocrine disorders

- Mental retardation associated with cranial abnormalities

- Mental retardation associated with genetic defects

Prenatal Factors

The term **prenatal** means *before birth*. Prenatal factors are those suffered by a pregnant woman which in turn cause fetal damage and associated mental retardation. There are many such factors, including the following:

Rubella (German measles): Even a slight maternal infection of rubella is sufficient to cause fetal damage. Infection during the first 10 weeks of pregnancy causes the greatest fetal damage and mental retardation. Hearing and visual handicaps also may be present. Speech and language delay are almost always present.

Prenatal lead poisoning: When a pregnant woman inhales lead fumes, the fetus may be damaged resulting in brain injury and mental retardation. This condition is noted in some factory workers who handle lead.

Mercury poisoning: When a pregnant woman inhales mercury fumes the fetus is affected. This results in poor physical and mental development.

Prenatal immunization: When a pregnant woman receives immunization shots for smallpox and similar diseases, the fetus may be affected.

Maternal anoxia: If a pregnant woman is anemic or suffers from vascular disorders that restrict the blood supply to the fetus, fetal damage could occur.

Prenatal trauma: Automobile and other kinds of accidents suffered by a pregnant woman, especially in the latter stages of pregnancy, are a frequent cause of fetal damage and mental retardation.

X-ray and radiation: When a pregnant woman is exposed to either excessive amounts of x-ray or radiation, fetal damage could result.

Prematurity and low birth weight: These two are often the result of many factors, most of them prenatal. Not all prematurely born infants and those born with low birth weight are mentally retarded; some may be, depending upon the extent of prematurity and underweight.

Fetal alcohol syndrome: Maternal alcoholism during pregnancy is now a known cause of fetal brain injury and mental retardation. Even social drinking during the early stages of pregnancy is a suspected cause of fetal brain injury.

Maternal drug abuse: Fetal exposure to various drugs because of maternal drug abuse is a frequent cause of mental retardation and associated health problems. Fetal exposure to crack cocaine has been a major factor.

UNIT NOTES

Natal Factors

Natal factors are those that are associated with birth. These factors affect the child during the process of birth and include the following:

Fetal anoxia: Prolonged labor and lack of crying soon after birth may reduce the oxygen supply to the brain of the newborn and may result in brain injury and mental retardation.

Other kinds of brain injury at birth: Many abnormal labor conditions including improper application of forceps, birth canal compression of the head, malpositions of the baby that result in prolonged labor may all cause brain injury and resulting mental retardation.

Postnatal Factors

Postnatal factors are those that come to play after the birth. In most cases, the child will have come in contact with some damaging chemical agent, including the following:

Post-immunization encephalitis: In some children, DPT immunization may cause an excessive reaction including high fever, convulsions, coma, slow recovery, and mental retardation. (D = Diphtheria; P = Pertussis or whooping cough; T = Tetanus or lockjaw.)

Rabies vaccine: In some children this may result in motor paralysis due to brain damage.

Lead poisoning or toxicity: Relatively rare, but very toxic (damaging to the nervous system). Children who have eaten peeled off paint from old buildings have suffered lead poisoning and brain damage.

Head Trauma

Head trauma is a frequent cause of brain injury and the consequent mental retardation. The variety of causes of head trauma include:

Vehicular accidents: Automobile accidents are a frequent cause of head trauma in children and adults. Bicycle and motorcycle accidents and off-road vehicular accidents also contribute greatly to the incidence of head trauma.

Other accidents: These include shocks applied to the head (shock therapy for individuals who are mentally ill), various industrial accidents, blast injuries, and other kinds of accidents.

Child abuse: Domestic violence and child abuse also are reported causes of head trauma.

Gunshot wounds: Victims of crime and gang violence are increasing in number in present-day society.

Metabolic Disorders

Metabolic disorders include many conditions, but two may be mentioned here:

Phenylketonuria (PKU): This occurs once in 10,000 births. Because of an absence of a liver enzyme, a chemical called phenylalanine is not metabolized. The resulting concentration of phenylalanine (an amino acid) in the body causes nerve and brain cell damage. The acid is detected in the urine. Most states require a test on all newborn babies to rule out PKU. The condition is effectively treated; therefore, the incidence of retardation due to PKU has declined.

Lipid metabolic errors: This is the presence of certain kinds of fat in neural cells. When the brain cells have those kinds of fat, the condition is called cerebral lipidosis. **Tay-Sachs disease,**

which is more frequently seen in Jewish children, is one such condition. The child is normal at birth but soon retardation becomes evident.

Endocrine Disorders

Among the endocrine disorders that are associated with retardation, the most notable is **hypothyroidism** (thyroid deficiency), which may have begun prenatally or postnatally. The child is subnormal in all functions including the heart rate, body temperature, blood pressure, respiration, and physical activity (which are all low). The child has a large, protruding tongue, dry and thick skin, and roundish face.

Cranial Abnormalities

Cranial abnormalities are congenital defects of the head and the skull. They may be due to toxic agents including maternal drug abuse, x-ray and radiation, vitamin deficiencies, chromosomal defects, and others. Among the more common cranial abnormalities are the following:

Anencephaly: This is the absence of cranial bones and often the cranial skin. The brain is exposed; sense organs may be missing; toxic agents are suspected; the child does not live for more than a few days.

Macrocephaly: The entire cranial vault is enlarged due to increase in the size of the brain (the cerebral hemispheres). The child has seizures along with mental retardation.

Hydrocephaly: This resembles macrocephaly, but it is due to a different cause. It is one of the most common cranial abnormalities. Spinal fluids, which do not flow as they normally do, get collected within the cranial vault. The head increases in size; intracranial pressure increases; eyes bulge out; the mental condition deteriorates rapidly. There is surgery to drain the fluid, but repeated surgeries often are needed; surgery itself can cause additional brain injury. There also are drugs that control the formation of the spinal fluids.

Microcephaly: The child is born with an extremely small head. This is due to lack of formation of brain tissue, especially that of the cerebral hemispheres.

Hereditary Factors and Genetic Syndromes

Genetic factors that cause mental retardation also are numerous. Many mild forms of mental retardation may be inherited. Inherited mental retardation is described as **familial**.

Among the many genetic syndromes that cause mental retardation, the following are often described in the literature:

Down syndrome: This syndrome is due to a chromosomal defect. While it is normal to have 46 chromosomes (23 pairs), the child with Down syndrome has 47 chromosomes; the small extra chromosome is the genetic defect that causes the syndrome.

Fragile X syndrome: This X-linked chromosomal abnormality is thought to cause the most common form of mental retardation in the male. The long arm of the X chromosome has a fragile site, hence the name.

Prader-Willie syndrome: Another genetic syndrome caused by chromosomal abnormality. In some cases, the abnormality is familial.

Cri Du Chat syndrome: In this syndrome, the short arm of the fifth chromosome is absent. The infant's cry sounds like that of a cat (hence the name).

UNIT NOTES

LANGUAGE DISORDERS OF CHILDREN WITH MENTAL RETARDATION

Whether the language of children with mental retardation is only quantitatively different from that of children who are nonretarded or if it also is qualitatively different has been debated. Mere **quantitative difference** suggests that children who are mentally retarded speak a language that is not unusual or bizarre, but simply limited. A child who is retarded may speak more like children of younger age who are nonretarded. For example, if a 10-year-old person who is retarded spoke more like a 4-year-old child, the language would not be considered qualitatively different.

A **qualitative difference** exists when persons who are retarded produce forms of language that are not heard in the population that is not retarded. Research has shown that some unusual expressions may be found in the language of persons who are profoundly retarded. However, for the most part, the language associated with mental retardation:

- is essentially simpler

- is limited in quantity

- follows the normal sequence

- is deficient in grammar

- is limited in social use

- is generally similar to the language of younger children

The language of the child who is retarded may be limited in every aspect, though the extent of the deficiency may depend upon the degree of retardation and the quality of special educational services offered and the age at which the child received them.

Phonological Aspects

The child who is retarded is likely to exhibit many errors of articulation. The child is likely to:

- omit, substitute, or distort speech sounds

- exhibit the same kinds of articulation problems as children who are not retarded

- use the same phonological processes as the nonretarded

Semantic Aspects of Language

Compared to children who are not retarded, those who are:

- acquire the first words later

- learn words more easily than syntactic structures

- learn new words at a slower rate, learn fewer words at a time

- have a smaller and more limited vocabulary

- have a less-varied, more concrete vocabulary

- use fewer adjectives and adverbs

Morphologic Aspects of Language

Morphologic features are frequently missing in the language of the child who is retarded. The child is likely to omit:

- the regular plural morpheme

- possessive inflections

- the present progressive *ing*

- the past tense inflection

- prepositions

- the auxiliary

and other morphologic features.

A point to remember is that on standardized tests of morphologic features, the child who is retarded does worse than in conversational speech. Therefore, it is better to use language samples than standardized tests in the assessment of the use of morphologic features in children who are retarded.

The child who is retarded follows the normal sequence in acquiring the morphological features.

Syntactic Aspects of Language

The child who is retarded:

- experiences difficulty in both understanding and producing various syntactic structures of language

- follows the normal sequence in mastering comprehension and production

- exhibits simpler syntactic structures

- uses less-varied syntactic structures

- shows limited elaborations

- uses fewer relative clauses

Generally, the higher the mental age, the more complex the sentence forms the child uses. Children who are profoundly retarded are either nonverbal, or if verbal, speak only in single words and gestures. Therefore, in such children, the syntactic skills may be mostly absent. The children in this group also tend to exhibit echolalia.

Pragmatic Aspects of Language

Pragmatic problems of children with retardation can be striking. The following problems often are noticed:

- reluctance to use the learned language skills in social situations

- difficulty in initiating conversation

- abrupt, short answers to questions

- responses that are inappropriate to time, place, and person

- problems in maintaining a topic of conversation with meaningful addition of new information

- inability to use conversational repair strategies (e.g., request for clarification)

- lack of appreciation of the listener's problems in understanding them (e.g., varying words or expressions)

- limited generalization of learned language skills

- deficient narrative skills

ASSOCIATED CONDITIONS

Children with mental retardation are likely to exhibit a variety of associated clinical conditions. The two that are most important are hearing loss and physical disabilities.

Hearing Loss

Hearing loss is more common in children who are retarded than in the general population. These children are prone to have **middle ear diseases** (such as otitis media) and accompanying **conductive hearing impairment**. Children with Down syndrome are especially prone to have middle ear infections and conductive hearing loss. Many diseases that are associated with mental retardation (such as rubella) also can damage the inner ear and the neural mechanism involved in hearing. Therefore, **sensorineural hearing loss** also is frequently observed in persons with retardation.

The presence of hearing loss in many children who are retarded may be partially responsible for some of the speech and language problems.

Physical Disabilities

Children with mental retardation are likely to have physical disabilities. They also are prone to frequent illnesses. Neurological impairment may be frequently observed.

TREATMENT OF LANGUAGE DISORDERS

Units 10 through 13 present language treatment and maintenance procedures. The same general principles of treatment apply to the teaching of language to children with mental retardation. Many treatment procedures also are the same across different populations of children with language disorders.

Here we take note of a few special considerations that apply to the treatment of language disorders in children with mental retardation. In treating such children, it is especially important to emphasize:

- training in more natural settings to promote generalization and appropriate use of language in everyday situations. If the treatment is started in a structured situation (the clinician's office, for example), it should soon be moved to other settings including playground, classroom, and home.

CLASS NOTES

- the use of objects and events instead of pictures as stimuli. The clinician can promote better generalization and maintenance if objects, especially those from the child's environment, are used as stimuli.

- shaping procedures in which a complex response is broken down into smaller components which are taught in graded steps and finally integrated.

- the use of modeling the correct responses for the child to imitate. The clinician's modeling must be withdrawn in gradual steps.

- immediate reinforcement of correct responses. In cases of children who are profoundly retarded, food and drink (primary reinforcers) may have to be used.

- expansion of utterances into grammatically more complete forms in natural settings and the reinforcement of expanded productions.

Efforts to teach oral communication skills to children who are profoundly retarded may fail. The clinician then may teach nonverbal means of communication. The use of sign language, communication boards, and other forms of nonverbal communication may be taught.

Instructor's Views and Critical Comments on the Language of Children Who Are Mentally Retarded

_____

_____

_____

_____

_____

_____

_____

_____

_____

_____

_____

_____

_____

_____

_____

_____

_____

_____

_____

_____

_____

REFERENCES AND READING ASSIGNMENTS

Grossman, H. J. (Ed.). (1983). *Classification in mental retardation.* Washington, DC: American Association on Mental Deficiency.

This is the standard manual for defining and classifying mental retardation.

Nelson, N. W. (1993). *Childhood language disorders in context.* New York: Macmillan.

Read Chapter 4 for a brief discussion of mental retardation and other conditions associated with language disorders.

Paul, R. (1995). *Language disorders from infancy through adolescence: Assessment and intervention.* St. Louis: Mosby.

Read the section on mental retardation in Chapter 5.

Reed, V. (1994). *An introduction to children with language disorders* (2nd ed.). New York: Macmillan.

Read Chapter 6 for details on mental retardation and language disorders.

Sparks, S. N. (1984). Speech and language in fetal alcohol syndrome. *Asha, 26,* 27–31.

Sprintzen, R. L., & Siegel-Sadewitz, V. L. (1982). The relationship of communication disorders in syndrome identification. *Journal of Speech and Hearing Disorders, 47,* 338–354.

Special Assignments From the Instructor:

_____

_____

_____

_____

_____

_____

_____

_____

_____

_____

_____

_____

_____

_____

_____

_____

_____

_____

_____

_____

_____

STUDY QUESTIONS

1. What is the definition of mental retardation given by the American Association on Mental Deficiency?

   _____

   _____

   _____

   _____

   _____

2. Describe a genetic cause of retardation that may have been environmentally induced:

   _____

   _____

   _____

   _____

   _____

3. Define the following terms:

   a. Prenatal: _____

   b. Natal: _____

   c. Postnatal _____

4. Describe three prenatal conditions that could be associated with mental retardation:

   _____

   _____

   _____

   _____

   _____

5. What are the two natal conditions associated with mental retardation?

   _____

   _____

   _____

   _____

6. What is post-immunization encephalitis?

_____

_____

_____

_____

7. What are some of the frequent causes of head trauma?

_____

_____

_____

_____

8. Describe PKU:

_____

_____

_____

_____

_____

9. What is hypothyroidism? What are its effects?

_____

_____

_____

_____

10. What is a lipid metabolic error?

_____

_____

_____

11. What is cerebral lipidosis?

_____

_____

_____

_____

12. What is Tay-Sachs disease?

_____

_____

_____

_____

13. Distinguish between macrocephaly and hydrocephaly:

_____

_____

_____

_____

14. What is the genetic basis of Down syndrome?

_____

_____

_____

_____

15. Distinguish between quantitative and qualitative differences in language behaviors exhibited by persons who are normal and those who are mentally retarded:

_____

_____

_____

_____

_____

16. Summarize the semantic aspects of the language of children with retardation:

_____

_____

_____

_____

_____

17. List the pragmatic problems children with retardation are likely to show:

_____

_____

_____

_____

_____

18. Specify a minimum of five sounds the children with retardation are likely to misarticulate: ____ ____ ____ ____ ____

19. Why should you train language behaviors in more natural settings?

_____

_____

_____

_____

20. In language treatment for children with retardation, why should you use objects and events instead of pictures?

_____

_____

_____

_____

21. What kinds of nonverbal modes of communication have been taught to persons who are retarded?

_____

_____

Autism and Language Disorders

- Characteristics of Children with Autism

- Theories of Autism

- Language Disorders Associated With Autism

- Treatment of Language Disorders

- References and Reading Assignments

- Study Questions

Leo Kanner, a child psychiatrist, originally described autism. For many years, autism was classified as a form of childhood psychosis.

Currently, experts think that autism is not a form of psychosis. Instead, they think that autism is a severe form of a **pervasive developmental disorder.**

The term autism is used to describe children who have most of the symptoms that characterize it. The term **autistic-like** is sometimes used to describe children who may show only some of the symptoms.

Autism affects 4 to 5 children in every 10,000. More males than females are affected, but female cases tend to be more severe.

Both verbal and nonverbal characteristics help identify autism. Multiple characteristics are necessary to make a diagnosis.

CHARACTERISTICS OF CHILDREN WITH AUTISM

According to the American Psychiatric Association's (1987) diagnostic criteria, autism has the following characteristics:

- Early onset. The early signs of autism are noticed during infancy or childhood

- Lack of responsiveness to people. The child may be unaware of others and their feelings

- No or abnormal (stereotypic) seeking of comfort when hurt or ill

- No or impaired imitation (echolalia)

- No or abnormal play

- No interest in making friends

- Lack of interest in communication (both verbal and nonverbal)

UNIT NOTES

- Abnormal nonverbal communication (lack of eye contact, stiffens when held)

- Absence of imaginative play

- Abnormal speech (high pitched, monotonous)

- Abnormal language (echolalia; idiosyncratic or irrelevant expressions)

- Difficulty in initiating and sustaining conversation

- Stereotypic body movements

- Preoccupation with objects or parts of objects

- Distress over changes in insignificant aspects of living

- Insistence on routines

- Limited interests and obsessive involvement with one or a few activities

Children with autism are disinterested in people, a major characteristic of the disorder. Aspects of this characteristic include the following:

- A preference for solitude and for objects rather than people

- Disinterest in the mother's voice

- Preference for mechanical noises

- Reluctance to be hugged, held, or even touched

- Tendency to walk away from people

- Preference to be left alone

One mother of an autistic daughter wrote: "She looked through human beings as if they were glass. She created solitude in the midst of company, silence in the midst of chatter" (Park, 1982, pp. 4–5).

In addition, some (not all) children with autism show:

- Self-injurious behaviors (e.g., banging their heads, chewing on their fingers, biting their own arms)

- Unusual talent in some areas (usually in arithmetic; excellent memory for numbers and fast arithmetic calculations)

Associated Problems

Other problems children with autism are likely to show include the following:

- Evidence of brain injury, especially damage to the left cerebral hemisphere

- Abnormal electrical activity of the brain

- Seizures

- Fragile X syndrome

- Hearing loss

- Hypo- or hypersensitivity to sensory stimuli

- Motor deficits

- Central auditory problems

- Mental retardation

THEORIES OF AUTISM

The causes of autism are not well understood. An early theory suggested that there may be a profound disturbance between the mother and the newborn baby. A failure to develop an emotional bonding between the mother and the baby was thought to cause autism. Most experts now disagree with this theory. Although there is a lack of emotional bonding between the baby and the mother, it may be an effect, not a cause, of autism.

Currently, most experts support genetic or neurophysiological theories of autism. Some believe that autism may have a genetic basis because of a slight hereditary tendency in its prevalence. However, no gene responsible for autism has been isolated. Other experts believe that brain injury may be the cause of autism.

LANGUAGE DISORDERS ASSOCIATED WITH AUTISM

The unique language of the child who is autistic is a significant diagnostic indicator.

The major characteristics of language and communication of children with autism include the following:

- Inadequate or lack of **response to speech**

- Slower acquisition of **speech sound production**

- Difficulty **producing speech sounds** correctly

- **Disinterest in communication** and meaningful exchange

- Lack of interest in **mother's voice**

- Better response to environmental **noises** than to human voices

- Better response to **pure tones** than to speech stimuli

- Fascination with **mechanical noises**

- Disinterest in **pointing** to things or **asking questions**

- Use of language in **stereotypic**, meaningless manner

- Slower **acquisition of language**

- More ready learning of **words that refer to objects** (*cup*, for example) rather than those that refer to human experiences and emotions (*love, hate, happy*) or those that refer to people (*Mommy, brother, sister*)

- Faster learning of **concrete words** than abstract words; however, some autistic children easily learn highly abstract words as long as they do not refer to human relations or emotions (e.g., one child could say words like *triangle* and *hexagon* but not *mommy, love,* or *hate*)

- Use of words in **restricted sense and contexts** (lack of generalized word meanings)

- Echolalic speech (**echolalia** is the parrot-like repetition of what others said; may be immediate or delayed; may echo TV commercials, words and phrases picked up from adult conversations; often not intended as communication, but there are some interesting exceptions)

- Lack of understanding of the **relation between words** (e.g., the relation between *needle* and *thread*, though they know the meaning of individual words)

- Use of **idiosyncratic metaphors** (unique expressions that reflect concreteness and bizarre restriction as well as unusual extension of word meaning)

- Difficulty in language **comprehension** (However, children who are autistic may recall meaningless words or sentences just as well as meaningful words and sentences)

- **Reversal of pronouns** (use of *you* for *I* and *I* for *you*; use of *he, she, him* or *her* to refer to themselves)

- Use of **simpler, shorter**, sentence structures

- Use of **wrong word order** in sentences

- **Omission of grammatic features** (e.g., auxiliaries, plural inflections, conjunctions, and prepositions)

- Use of **inappropriate language** (inappropriate to time, place, and person)

- Lack of eye contact

- Lack of topic maintenance in conversation

and other pragmatic problems

Though appearing engrossed, children who are autistic repeat what someone said months ago, suggesting they do pay some attention to speech around them.

Some of the echolalic responses may be an attempt at communication because such responses include an answer to the question asked. One child for example, who was asked "What do you want?" replied "What do you want candy" (echolalia plus the child's response).

TREATMENT OF LANGUAGE DISORDERS

Units 10 through 13 present language treatment procedures, variations, and maintenance. Many of the general principles and procedures of language treatment also are used in treating children with autism. Here, a few special concerns or procedures are highlighted:

- Use **objects** rather than pictorial stimuli in teaching words; because children who are autistic respond better to concrete objects than to pictures.

- Teach words and other elements of language in a **variety of contexts** and environmental situations so that the child does not use words in restricted senses and contexts.

- Use the widely researched **behavioral principles** in treating language problems of children with autism.

- Teach **alternative responses** that replace echolalia; see if language responses can be built upon the existing echolalia.

- **Reduce pronoun reversal** by referring to the child by his or her proper name.

- Use **direct, intensive training** for children with severe autistic behaviors.

- Pay particular attention to **generalization and maintenance strategies** as children with autism do not readily generalize or maintain learned responses.

- Consider **nonverbal methods of communication** when intensive and prolonged attempts at teaching oral communication fail; children who are autistic are known to learn signs with relative ease.

- Consult with **other specialists** and make sure the child is referred to specialists whose services are needed.

Instructor's Views and Critical Comments on Language of Children With Autism _____

_____

_____

_____

_____

_____

_____

_____

_____

_____

_____

_____

_____

_____

_____

_____

_____

_____

_____

_____

_____

_____

_____

REFERENCES AND READING ASSIGNMENTS

American Psychiatric Association. (1987). *Diagnostic and statistical manual of mental disorders* (3rd ed. revised). Washington, DC: Author.

Consult this standard manual for psychiatric diagnostic categories.

Nelson, N. W. (1993). *Childhood language disorders in context.* New York: Macmillan.

Read Chapter 4 for a brief discussion of autism and other conditions

Paul, R. (1995). *Language disorders from infancy through adolescence: Assessment and intervention.* St. Louis: Mosby.

Read the section on autism in Chapter 5.

Park, C. C. (1982). *The siege.* Boston: Little, Brown & Company.

Read this book for a fascinating account of autism written by a mother whose daughter was autistic.

Reed, V. (1994). *An introduction to children with language disorders* (2nd ed.). New York: Macmillan.

Read Chapter 8 for details on autism and language disorders.

Special Assignments From the Instructor:

_____

_____

_____

_____

_____

_____

_____

_____

_____

_____

_____

_____

_____

_____

_____

_____

_____

_____

_____

_____

_____

_____

_____

STUDY QUESTIONS

1. Who first described autism? _____

2. How common is autism in the general population?

    _____

3. Who are autistic-like children? How do they differ from children with autism?

    _____

    _____

    _____

4. List the major symptoms of autism:

    _____

    _____

    _____

    _____

    _____

    _____

    _____

    _____

    _____

    _____

5. List the problems associated with autism:

    _____

    _____

    _____

    _____

6. List the major characteristics of the language of children with autism::

    _____

    _____

    _____

    _____

_____

_____

_____

_____

7. Describe the kinds of words children with autism learn more readily:

_____

_____

8. What is echolalia? What are the two kinds of echolalia?

_____

_____

_____

9. Give an example of lack of understanding of the relation between words that children with autism exhibit:

_____

_____

10. What is pronoun reversal? Give examples:

_____

_____

_____

11. What kinds of grammatic features are likely to be missing in the speech of children who are autistic? Be specific and give examples:

_____

_____

_____

_____

12. Give an example of echolalia that may be an attempt at communication:

_____

_____

_____

13. What kinds of stimuli would you use in teaching words to children who are autistic?

_____

14. Why should you teach words in a variety of contexts and situations?

_____

_____

15. When do you consider teaching nonverbal communication for children who are autistic?

_____

_____

_____

16. To what other specialists would you consider referring a child with autism?

_____

_____

_____

Hearing Impairment and Language Disorders

UNIT NOTES

In this Unit, you will learn about language disorders exhibited by children with hearing impairment.

HEARING AND LANGUAGE

A strong relation between normal hearing and normal oral language acquisition is well established. Normal hearing is essential for oral language acquisition and production because of two important reasons. First, normal hearing makes the child aware of the spoken language. Second, normal hearing makes it possible to self-monitor language production. The child can listen not only to the speech of other persons, but also to his or her own speech and modify it to match the adult model.

In the absence of normal hearing, the child is not fully aware of what needs to be learned, and whatever is learned and produced is not fully self-monitored. These two problems create the variety of communicative disorders exhibited by persons with hearing impairment. Hearing impairment causes not only language acquisition problems, but also problems of speech production (articulation), voice, resonance, fluency, rate, and rhythm. Finally, hearing impairment makes it difficult to comprehend spoken language.

DEFINITION OF BASIC TERMS

Hearing impairment and **hearing loss** are general terms that suggest a hearing problem. The terms mean that the individual's auditory system is not functioning normally and the auditory thresholds exceed 25 dBHL in the case of adults and 15 dB in the case of children.

Hard of hearing means that the person has a hearing problem but still is able to use his or her hearing for speech-language acquisition, comprehension, and production. A hard of hearing person is aware of normal conversational speech; the person, however, may need amplification.

Deaf means that an individual is not aware of normal conversation and is not able to use his or her hearing for speech-language acquisition, comprehension, and production.

Acquired hearing loss has an onset subsequent to birth; it is not congenital.

Congenital hearing loss is present at the time of birth.

Hearing acuity means how well a person hears and it is measured in terms of decibels (dB).

The **range of normal hearing** varies from 0 dBHL to 15 dBHL (children) and 0 dBHL to 25 dBHL (adults).

The **severity of hearing impairment** may be rated as follows:

• Slight impairment: 16 to 25 dBHL

• Mild impairment: 26 to 40 dBHL

• Moderate impairment: 41 to 70 dBHL

• Severe impairment: 71 to 90 dBHL

• Profound impairment: 91+ dBHL

Remember that hearing loss itself is on a *continuum* and such rating categories are arbitrary. Two persons, one with 70 dBHL loss and another with 71 dBHL loss, may be placed in different categories, but such categorization may not be clinically meaningful; their communicative skills may be more similar than different.

Review an audiology textbook to learn more about hearing loss, its various pathologies, and aural rehabilitation (Alpiner & McCarthy, 1993; Martin, 1994; Northern & Downs, 1991).

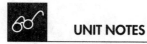

FACTORS THAT AFFECT THE COMMUNICATIVE BEHAVIORS

Hearing impairment produces varied effects across children. Factors that contribute to such individual differences include the following:

The age of onset: Generally, the earlier the onset, the greater the negative effects on language acquisition and production. Congenital hearing impairment produces the greatest effects. Hearing loss acquired after language learning is completed produces less severe effects.

The degree of loss: Generally, the greater the loss, the more profound the effects on communicative skills.

It was believed years ago that a mild hearing loss that often accompanies middle ear infection does not produce much of an effect on speech and language acquisition. Recent research suggests that even a loss in the range of 15–25 dB may be sufficient to cause delay in speech and language acquisition.

The age of onset and the degree of loss interact: The earlier the onset and the greater the loss, the more profound the effects; the later the onset and the milder the loss, the lesser the effects.

Age of detection of hearing loss: The sooner the hearing loss is detected, the better it is for the child because early intervention becomes possible. The earlier the intervention, the greater the chances for better communicative skills. Generally, it is the mild and moderate degrees of hearing losses that go unnoticed until school age. Severe to profound losses are more readily detected at an early age.

The presence of other handicapping conditions: When hearing loss is associated with mental retardation, neurological impairment, and visual problems, the negative effects on communicative skills are greater.

CLASS NOTES

The types of auditory pathology and hearing loss: Generally, conductive hearing loss produces less severe effects than the sensorineural loss. This is so because conductive losses are less severe and more readily managed with amplification and medical means than are sensorineural losses.

The age at which intervention is started: The earlier the onset of language intervention, the greater the oral language skills of a child who is hearing impaired.

LANGUAGE AND SPEECH PROBLEMS OF CHILDREN WITH HEARING IMPAIRMENT

What follows is a general list of language and speech problems of children who are hearing impaired; it is assumed that the degree of loss is significant enough to produce negative effects. Please remember that the extent of the problems a given child exhibits depends upon the variables described previously.

Morphologic and Syntactic Problems

The morphologic and syntactic behaviors of children who are hard of hearing are minimally affected, but those of children who are deaf are maximally affected. The following are the typical effects of hearing impairment:

• **Slower acquisition** of morphologic and syntactic structures.

• **Omission of morphologic features** in conversational speech resulting in telegraphic speech (e.g., omission or inconsistent production of articles, prepositions, conjunctions, past tense inflections, the regular plural inflections, the present progressive, and the third person singular).

• Difficulty understanding or producing **complex, compound,** and **embedded sentences**.

Semantic Problems

Children who are hearing impaired show the following kinds of semantic problems:

- **Limited vocabulary** lacking in both quantity and variety.

- **Poor comprehension** of word meanings.

- **Restricted use of word meanings** in sentences produced.

- **Failure to understand multiple meanings** of words. Persons who are hearing impaired may only understand one or two meanings that are commonly associated with words.

- **Failure to understand abstract, metaphoric**, and **proverbial phrases** and **sentences**. Persons who are hearing impaired interpret such phrases and sentences literally.

Pragmatic Problems

Persons who are hearing impaired may not know how to use the learned language in natural social situations. The following pragmatic communication problems are likely:

- **Reluctance to speak:** Even when they can, some persons with hearing problems may not speak.

- **Limited communication:** Persons with hearing impairment may not say enough, answer strictly to the point, and elaborate on what they say. They may not give sufficient background information on what they say.

- **Inappropriate speech:** The speech of some persons with hearing impairment also may be inappropriate to the situation or topic of discussion.

UNIT NOTES

CLASS NOTES

Speech Production Problems

Individuals with hearing impairment tend to exhibit numerous errors of articulation, including the following:

- **Omission** of consonants at the end of words and in blends

- **Substitution** of voiced consonants for voiceless and vice versa

- **Greater difficulty** in the correct production of **fricatives** (*s, z, sh*, and *th*) and **affricates** (*ch* and *j*)

- **Distortions** of various sounds

- **Nasal resonance** on nonnasal sounds (hypernasality)

- **Reduced nasal resonance** on nasal sounds (hyponasality)

- **Omission of sounds** that are produced at the back of the oral cavity (*g, k*)

Other Communication Problems

Other problems persons with hearing impairment experience include problems of voice, rhythm, and fluency:

- **Voice quality problems**, noted mostly in individuals who are deaf (not in individuals who are hard of hearing) include high pitch, nasality, lack of pitch and loudness variations, harshness, and hoarseness

- A **slower rate of speech** (halting speech with slow delivery)

- **Abnormal flow of speech** where speech may lack the normal rhythm

CLASS NOTES

• **Limited fluency**, due mostly to limited language skills and production problems

LANGUAGE TREATMENT

Units 10 through 13 present information on language treatment, variations, and maintenance. Once again, note here that the general principles of treatment apply across children who exhibit language disorders regardless of associated conditions such as mental retardation or hearing impairment. Even many of the treatment procedures also will be similar across different groups of children with language disorders.

The following are a few unique aspects of the language treatment for children who are hearing impaired:

• **Early identification** of hearing loss is critical. The presence of such factors as the family history of hearing loss, administration of ototoxic drugs, craniofacial anomalies, congenital infections are warning signals (ASHA, 1991).

• **Early medical management** is important in case of children with middle ear infections.

• **Early audiological management**, including the use of amplification and aural rehabilitation, is essential.

• **Early oral language intervention** also is critical for success in acquiring oral language.

• **Multiple services** that the child needs must be provided as early as possible (psychological, educational, social, medical, and other services).

• **Words, morphologic aspects, syntactic structures**, and **pragmatic use of language** are all appropriate treatment targets.

• **Parent involvement** in the educational process is important. The parents and other family members should be trained to reinforce the production of

UNIT NOTES

CLASS NOTES

correct communicative behaviors at home and other natural settings.

• **Use of visual cues** in teaching is essential during language training.

• **Use of group or personal FM hearing amplification systems** may be helpful.

• **Nonverbal means of communication**, including American Sign Language (ASL) may be appropriate. Speech-language pathologists who cannot teach ASL or other forms of nonverbal communication should make appropriate referrals.

Instructor's Views and Critical Comments on Language of Children with Hearing Impairment _____

_____

_____

_____

_____

_____

_____

_____

_____

_____

_____

_____

_____

_____

_____

_____

_____

_____

_____

_____

_____

_____

_____

REFERENCES AND READING ASSIGNMENTS

Alpiner J. G., & McCarthy, P. A. (1993). *Rehabilitative audiology: Children and adults.* Baltimore: Williams & Wilkins.

Use this as your resourcebook on aural rehabilitation.

ASHA (1991). Joint Committee on Infant Hearing 1990 position statement. *Asha, 33,* (Suppl. 5), 3–6.

Kelly, B. R., Davis, D., & Hegde, M. N. (1994). *Clinical methods and practicum in audiology.* San Diego: Singular Publishing Group.

Parts II through IV contain audiological management of persons with hearing impairment. Use this as a resource book.

Martin, F. N. (1994). *Introduction to audiology* (5th ed.). Englewood Cliffs, NJ: Prentice-Hall.

You may use this as one of your reference books on audiology.

Nelson, N. W. (1993). *Childhood language disorders in context.* New York: Macmillan.

Read Chapter 4 for a discussion of hearing impairment and other conditions.

Northern, J. L., & Downs, M. P. (1991). *Hearing in children* (4th ed.). Baltimore: Williams & Wilkins.

You may use this as one of your reference books on pediatric audiology.

Reed, V. (1994). *An introduction to children with language disorders* (2nd ed.). New York: Macmillan.

Read Chapter 9 for details on autism and language disorders.

Special Assignments From the Instructor:

_____

_____

_____

_____

_____

_____

_____

_____

_____

_____

_____

_____

_____

_____

_____

_____

_____

_____

_____

_____

_____

STUDY QUESTIONS

1. State the two reasons why hearing impairment causes speech-language problems:

   1. _____

   _____

   2. _____

   _____

2. Define the following terms:

   (a) A person with hearing loss or impairment

   _____

   _____

   _____

   (b) Hard of hearing

   _____

   _____

   _____

   (c) Deaf

   _____

   _____

   _____

   (d) Acquired hearing loss

   _____

   _____

   (e) Congenital hearing loss

   _____

   _____

   _____

(f) The range of normal hearing:

For children _____

For adults _____

(g) The dBHL ranges for:

slight loss_____; mild loss: _____

moderate loss_____; severe loss _____

profound loss_____.

3. What is the limitation of the hearing loss rating categories?

_____

_____

_____

4. List the six major factors that affect the communicative behaviors of the hearing impaired:

1. _____ 2. _____

3. _____ 4. _____

5. _____ 6. _____

5. How do the age of onset and the degree of loss interact?

_____

_____

_____

6. Summarize the morphologic problems of children who are hearing impaired:

_____

_____

_____

7. Summarize the syntactic problems of children who are hearing impaired:

_____

_____

_____

8. What is telegraphic speech?

_____

_____

9. Why do children with hearing impairment find it difficult to learn morphologic features?

_____

_____

10. Summarize the semantic problems of children who are hearing impaired:

_____

_____

_____

_____

11. Give an example of a metaphoric or proverbial expression that is difficult for the person with hearing impairment to comprehend. State how the person might interpret your example.

_____

_____

_____

_____

12. Give an example for "a failure to understand the multiple meanings of a word":

_____

_____

_____

_____

13. Summarize the pragmatic problems of persons who are hearing impaired:

_____

_____

_____

14. List the sounds the persons with hearing impairment are likely to misarticulate:

_____

_____

15. Describe the voice qualities of a person who is deaf:

_____

_____

_____

_____

16. List the major risk factors for hearing impairment in infants:

_____

_____

_____

_____

17. What kinds of stimuli and cues would you prefer in teaching language to children with hearing impairment?

_____

18. What is a wireless FM amplification system?

_____

_____

_____

_____

Brain Injury and Language Disorders

UNIT NOTES

In this Unit, you will learn about children whose language problems are a result of brain injury. Neurological involvement may be accompanied by other physical and sensory disabilities. If they are, the child is severely affected.

The children described in this unit consist of different subgroups. They often are classified in different ways: Physically disabled, neurologically involved, cerebral palsied, and traumatically brain injured are among the descriptions that can be applied to children in this group. The children show varied symptoms in the subgroups. A central problem of all of these children is some form of brain injury, though suffered at different times in their lives.

There are many causes of brain injury. These causes may operate at different periods of time including the prenatal, natal, and postnatal periods. In most cases, communication is affected.

Approximately 4% of children in kindergarten through the 12th grade may suffer from brain injury. Up to 20% of children receiving special education services may have suffered brain injury. More boys than girls experience brain injury.

CAUSES OF BRAIN INJURY

Among the many causes, the following are more common:

- **Vehicular accidents** in which the injured may be a passenger, pedestrian, driver, or bicycle rider. With adolescent drivers, car accidents are the major cause of brain injury.

- **Sports related accidents** involve motorcycle or dirtbike racing, skateboard riding, skiing, and other sport activities.

- **Falls** are a common cause of brain injury in children under age 2.

- **Physical abuse** is a significant cause of brain injury and the frequency is probably higher than reported.

- **Assault and gunshots** are a major cause in certain neighborhoods and big cities; adolescents are the common victims.

TRAUMATIC BRAIN INJURY

Traumatic brain injury is cerebral damage due to external physical force. The injury is not congenital nor is it a result of neurological disease. Depending on the severity of the external force, the injury may be minimal or extensive; focal or diffuse.

Focal injury is restricted to an area of the brain.

Diffuse injury involves multiple areas because the tissue damage is widespread.

In **nonpenetrating brain injury, meninges are intact,** but the skull may be intact or fractured. Nonpenetrating brain injury also is described as **closed-head injury.**

In **penetrating brain injury, the meninges are torn or lacerated.** The skull is perforated or fractured. Penetrating brain injuries also are known as **open-head injuries.**

Head injury and brain injury are not the same. There may be minor head injuries that do not injure the brain.

Coup injury is injury at the point of impact. This occurs when a head, because it receives a blow or rapidly moves and hits an object (as in auto accidents), causes the brain to move and slam against the point of impact.

Contrecoup injury is injury at the opposite side of the impact. This occurs when the brain that moved and slammed against the skull on the side of impact now moves back and slams against the opposite side.

Stretching of the brain tissue is the result of rotational forces that act on the brain.

Abrasion is laceration or tearing of tissue. This occurs when the brain moves back and forth on the surface of the skull which contains rough projections that tear the tissue.

EFFECTS OF TRAUMATIC BRAIN INJURY

Immediate effects include the following:

- **Coma.** This is loss of consciousness that lasts for longer intervals (an hour or more).

- **Slow or rapid recovery** from coma. The period immediately following recovery from coma is called the **acute recovery period**.

- **Confusion and post-traumatic amnesia.** These are evident following the recovery from coma. Amnesia (loss of memory) is especially serious for recent events.

- **Retrograde amnesia**, which is difficulty in remembering the events leading to the traumatic episode.

- **Abnormal behaviors** including irritability, aggression, anxiety, and hyperactivity as well as lethargy, and withdrawal.

- **Motor dysfunctions** including rigidity, tremors, spasticity, ataxia, or apraxia may be present.

Language and Communication Disorders

The **Initial effects** (observed during the acute recovery period) include the following:

- **Mutism** and **speech production problems**. Difficulty in producing consonants may be pronounced. Soon the child may recover from these effects.

- **Speech comprehension problems**. These problems are variable, but the children experience greater difficulty comprehending sentences than words.

- **Word retrieval problems**. Difficulty may be more pronounced for words in certain categories.

- **Syntactic problems**. Limited MLU, fewer utterances, difficulty constructing sentences or describing objects may be present.

- **Writing problems**. These may be more serious than speaking problems.

Some of these initial effects may persist to some extent.

Long-term or residual effects include the following:

- **Reduction in spontaneous speech**.

- **Persistent word retrieval problems**. This may lead to indirect and imprecise expressions.

- **Reduced fluency** because of word retrieval problems.

- **Pragmatic problems** including difficulty in turn taking and topic maintenance.

- **Subtle comprehension problems** that become evident in demanding situations.

Experts now believe that children's level of recovery from the effects of brain injury has been exaggerated. Children continue to experience long-term effects (Ylvisaker, 1985).

Other Persistent Problems

- Poor academic performance

- Poor writing skills

- Reading problems

UNIT NOTES

- Impaired mathematical reasoning skills

- Memory problems

- Hyperactivity and impulsivity

- Inability to recognize their difficulties

STROKES AND BRAIN TUMORS IN CHILDREN

Besides traumatic brain injury, vascular and neurological diseases also can cause language disorders, resulting in aphasia.

Aphasia is a language disorder that results from brain injury whose most frequent cause is a stroke. **Strokes**, also known as **cerebrovascular accidents**, are more frequent in adults than in children.

Causes of strokes include:

- **Blocked arteries** that restrict blood supply to a part of the brain because of:

  - **cerebral thrombosis** (formation of a blood clot due to **arteriosclerosis**)

  - **embolism** (obstruction of blood flow by a traveling blood clot or foreign material)

- **Ruptured blood vessels** that cause brain **hemorrhage** (e.g., ruptured aneurysm which is balloon-like malformation of an artery which bursts under high and varying blood pressure)

Brain tumors also can cause aphasia; these, too, are more frequent in adults than in children.

  - **primary tumors** are those that have grown in the brain itself

  - **metastatic tumors** are those that have grown elsewhere in the body but have migrated to the brain where they continue to grow

Children who become aphasic because of strokes or tumors recover better than adults who have the same problem. However, recent opinion is that the extent of recovery has been overstated. Residual symptoms are more common than previously thought.

Most children exhibit **nonfluent aphasia**, which is characterized by:

- **Mutism** immediately following brain injury

- **Sparse** and **effortful** speech

- **Impaired repetition** of speech

- **Syntactic problems**

- **Auditory comprehension** problems

- **Anomia** (naming difficulties)

- **Reading** problems

- **Writing** problems

Aphasia in children is less likely to show:

- **Paraphasia** (unintended word or sound substitutions)

- **Jargon** (meaningless words the patient creates)

- **Fluent aphasia** (flowing but meaningless speech), which are all seen in adult patients

A Note on Developmental Aphasia

This term refers to children who have language disorders in the absence of hearing loss, mental retardation, autism, neurological involvement, or behavioral and emotional disorders. In essence, when nothing else explains the disorder, it may be developmental aphasia. However, the diagnostic category of developmental aphasia is controversial and many experts question its existence. Most now prefer the term **specific language impairment** described in Unit 2. As noted there, this newer term, too, is controversial.

TREATMENT OF LANGUAGE DISORDERS ASSOCIATED WITH BRAIN INJURY

Treatment of language disorders in children is presented in Units 10 through 13. Here, some special considerations that apply to treating children with brain injury are presented.

Assessment

Make a careful assessment of the child's needs, residual strengths, and weaknesses

- Make an assessment of family involvement, strengths, and needs

- Make an assessment of speech and language skills and problems

- Consider the educational, emotional, and social needs of the child

- Design a treatment plan based on the assessment results

Treatment Strategies

- **Family counseling:** During the acute phase, the family is counseled regarding the potential for regaining speech and general strategies of communication with the individual with brain injury.

- **Team involvement** in treatment planning and implementation. Treatment is typically managed by a multidisciplinary team.

- **Brief treatment sessions:** The session durations initially will be brief and they may be increased gradually.

- **Functional communication.** This is the initial target. Refinement of skills is for later stages of intervention.

- **Targeting dominant problems.** Whether they are word retrieval problems or speech production problems, the dominant problems are first targeted for remediation.

- **Treatment of motor speech disorders.** This is undertaken as the assessment results warrant their treatment.

- **Pragmatic communication skills.** The approach should be naturalistic communication.

- **Use of nonverbal communication methods.** Use them with caution, and only when justified.

- **Work with educators.** Facilitating the child's entry to school is an important part of treatment.

Consult other sources for additional information on traumatic brain injury in children and adolescents (Bigler, 1990; Mira, Tucker, & Tyler, 1992; Ylvisaker, 1985).

CEREBRAL PALSY

Palsy is paralysis. Cerebral palsy is a disorder of early childhood in which the immature nervous system is affected resulting in muscular incoordination and associated problems.

The origin may have been **prenatal** because in most cases, the disorder is **congenital** (noticed at the time or soon after birth). Cerebral palsy is not a progressive disease; most children improve as they grow older. Cerebral palsy is not the name of a disease; it describes certain effects.

Causes of Cerebral Palsy

There are many causes of cerebral palsy (CP); most are environmental factors that cause brain injury; most were described in Unit 4 on mental retardation.

• **Prenatal brain injury** due to:

maternal rubella, mumps, influenza, anemia resulting in fetal anoxia, Rh incompatibility, x-ray and radiation, anesthesia, and automobile and other accidents.

• **Natal brain injury** due to:

prolonged labor, breach delivery, and prematurity.

• **Postnatal brain injury** due to:

anoxia; automobile accidents; infections and diseases including mumps, scarlet fever, measles, whooping cough, meningitis, and encephalitis; lead and mercury poisoning.

Types of Cerebral Palsy

One classification is based on the **body parts that are paralyzed:**

Hemiplegia: Only one side of the body (either the left or the right side) is paralyzed.

Paraplegia: Only the legs and lower part of the body (lower trunk) are paralyzed; the arms are not involved.

Monoplegia: Only one limb (extremity) or a part is paralyzed.

Diplegia: Either the legs or the arms are paralyzed (but not both). This is bilateral paralysis (paralysis of corresponding parts on both sides of the body).

Quadriplegia: All four limbs are paralyzed.

Another classification has three major types:

Spastic CP: The most common type; increased **spasticity** (increased tone, rigidity) of the muscles; and jerky, slow, abrupt, stiff muscle movements because opposing muscles are simultaneously active. Cause is damage to the **motor cortex** or **direct motor pathways.**

Athetoid CP: Slow, involuntary, writhing, and worm-like movements are called **athetosis**. Cause is damage to **indirect motor pathways**, especially to the **basal ganglia.**

Ataxic CP: Disturbed balance, awkward gait, clumsy and uncoordinated movements characterize **ataxia**. Cause is damage to the cerebellum.

Abnormal reflexes are a major problem of children with cerebral palsy. In addition, these children have many associated problems including orthopedic abnormalities, seizures, feeding difficulties, hearing loss, perceptual disturbances, and intellectual deficits. Not all children with cerebral palsy have all of these problems, however. For example, some of them have normal or superior intelligence.

Speech and Language Problems Associated with Cerebral Palsy

Language acquisition in many children with CP is delayed. The extent of the delay is greater if the child also suffers from one or more of the associated problems (hearing loss, mental retardation). If the child has no other problem, the delay may be minimal.

The most significant problem associated with the CP is speech production. Because of the paralysis or weakness of the muscles of speech, articulation is almost always affected. Such muscle weakness or paralysis not only affects articulation, but also respiration, phonation, resonance, fluency, and prosody (intonation and rhythm). Such a cluster of speech disorders that are due to muscle paralysis (defective neural control of the muscles) is called **dysarthria**.

Language Treatment for Children with Cerebral Palsy

A generally applicable language treatment program, procedural variations, and maintenance are presented in Units 10 through 13. Therefore, a few special considerations of treatment of children with cerebral palsy are highlighted here.

The rehabilitation of children with cerebral palsy is a team effort involving:

• Speech-language pathologists

• Audiologists

• Otologists

• Neurologists

• Orthopedic surgeons

• Physical therapists

• Psychologists

• Social workers

• Special education specialists

The need for language intervention must be carefully assessed. The language treatment follows the same general principles of teaching **basic vocabulary** first and then, in graded steps, **phrases** and **sentences**. In most cases, the clinician is likely to spend more time teaching correct articulation than language.

Some profoundly involved children, especially those who are multiply handicapped (mental retardation and hearing impairment along with CP) may not be able to learn oral language. These children are candidates for nonverbal or alternative means of communication, described in the next section.

UNIT NOTES

ALTERNATIVE METHODS OF COMMUNICATION

Alternative methods of communication are useful for any child or adult whose potential for oral communication is limited. Children with severe cerebral palsy, profound mental retardation, physical disabilities, deafness, severe brain injury, and so forth are candidates for nonverbal means of communication.

Assessment of Children Who are Nonverbal

Careful assessment is needed to determine the strengths and limitations of the child:

- Make a client-specific assessment

- Assess the potential for oral communication

- Assess motor capabilities to select intervention strategies

- Assess sensory capabilities that dictate treatment options

- Assess the communication needs and demands placed on the child

- Assess educational needs

- Assess the adaptive strategies the child already has mastered

- Assess family support and involvement

Treatment Approaches for Nonverbal Children

There are different modes of nonverbal communication; depending on the assessment, one of the following may be selected for the child:

Manual modes of communication. This includes the widely used American Sign Language (ASL). It often is the dominant mode of communication for the deaf. However, any type of manual communication may pose special difficulties for children with cerebral palsy whose hands are paralyzed. Most manual modes require a certain degree of motor control and coordination. In fact, manual signing and manual alphabet require a high degree of fine motor coordination.

Communication boards and symbolic Communication. Individuals who cannot use their hands for signs or gestures can communicate with the help of a board which contains words, various preselected messages, and symbols. The child who can read but cannot talk (because of the paralysis of the speech muscles) may point to the words or even form simple sentences by pointing to words in sequence. A stick attached to the head may be used to point.

Children who cannot read may point to symbols that stand for words and actions. The symbols may be:

Abstract, geometric shapes. Specific word meanings are then attached to them by training. The Carrier symbols are an example.

Iconic symbols or pictures. These look like the objects they represent.

Blissymbolics. It was developed by Charles Bliss and has been used in teaching communicative skills to children with cerebral palsy. Some of the Blissymbols are semi-iconic, others are abstract shapes. The symbols are placed on a board along with words below them. The child *talks* by pointing to the symbols and the *listener* understands by reading the words under the symbols pointed out.

Rebus system. A rebus is a picture of an object or a person; it is iconic.

Computerized systems. These help generate messages on the computer monitor when operated by the person who is nonverbal. A person who is paralyzed, for example, can generate a message by a mere eyeblink. Electronic switches of various kinds that can be used to generate messages include pads, switches, and plates that may be touched; wobble sticks (joy sticks), squeeze bulbs, foot switches, and pneumatic switches that are activated by blowing or sucking; sound switches that are activated by sound, and so forth.

Instructor's Views and Critical Comments on Language of Children with Brain Injury _____

_____

_____

_____

_____

_____

_____

_____

_____

_____

_____

_____

_____

_____

_____

_____

_____

_____

_____

_____

_____

REFERENCES AND READING ASSIGNMENTS

Bigler, E. (Ed.). (1990). *Traumatic brain injury*. Austin, TX: PRO-ED.

Use this as a resource on rehabilitation of individuals with traumatic brain injury.

Mira, M. P., Tucker, B. F., & Taylor, J. S. (1992). *Traumatic brain injury in children and adolescents: A sourcebook for teachers and other school personnel*. Austin, TX: PRO-ED.

Read this simplified presentation of information on traumatic brain injury in children and adolescents.

Nelson, N. W. (1993). *Childhood language disorders in context*. New York: Macmillan.

Read the section on *Physical Impairment and Speech Motor Control* in Chapter 4.

Reed, V. (1994). *An introduction to children with language disorders* (2nd ed.). New York: Macmillan.

Read Chapter 12 on children with acquired language disorders.

Ylvisaker, M. (Ed.). (1985). *Head injury rehabilitation*. Austin, TX: PRO-ED.

Read chapters in this book on assessment and rehabilitation of children with brain injury.

Special Assignments From the Instructor:

_____

_____

_____

_____

_____

_____

_____

_____

_____

_____

_____

_____

_____

_____

_____

_____

_____

_____

_____

_____

_____

STUDY QUESTIONS

1. List the causes of brain injury:

   _____   _____

   _____   _____

   _____   _____

2. Define the following terms:

   a. Traumatic brain injury

   _____

   _____

   b. Nonpenetrating brain injury

   _____

   _____

   c. Penetrating brain injury

   _____

   _____

   d. Coup and contrecoup injuries

   _____

   _____

   _____

   _____

   e. Abrasion

   _____

   _____

   f. Retrograde amnesia

   _____

   _____

   _____

3. Describe the initial language problems associated with traumatic brain injury:

_____

_____

_____

_____

_____

_____

_____

4. Describe the long-term language problems associated with traumatic brain injury:

_____

_____

_____

_____

_____

_____

_____

_____

5. Define the following terms:

a. Aphasia

_____

_____

b. Cerebral thrombosis

_____

_____

c. Embolism

_____

_____

d. Arteriosclerosis

_____

_____

e. Metastatic tumors

_____

_____

f. Anomia

_____

_____

g. Paraphasia

_____

_____

6. What is cerebral palsy?

_____

_____

_____

_____

7. What are four potential causes of CP?

1. _____   2. _____

3. _____   4. _____

8. Define the following terms:

a. Hemiplegia

_____

b. Paraplegia

_____

c. Monoplegia

_____

d. Diplegia

_____

e. Quadriplegia

_____

9. Briefly describe spastic, athetoid, and ataxic CP. Specify the brain areas that are injured:

_____

_____

_____

_____

_____

10. Who are some of the specialists on a team that handles the rehabilitation of children with cerebral palsy?

_____

_____

_____

11. Who are the appropriate candidates for nonverbal communication?

_____

_____

12. When do you decide to teach a nonverbal mode of communication to a child?

_____

_____

13. What is a widely used manual mode of communication?

_____

14. List the steps you would take in assessing a nonverbal child:

_____

_____

_____

_____

_____

_____

15. Define the following terms:

a. Iconic symbols

_____

_____

b. Carrier symbols

_____

_____

c. Blissymbolics

_____

_____

d. A rebus

_____

_____

Cultural Diversity and Language Disorders

Cultural and linguistic diversity affects assessment and treatment of language disorders in children. As the United States has become more diversified both ethnically and linguistically, the issue of how to offer the most appropriate speech-language services to a diverse population has received much attention in recent years. Therefore, in this Unit, you will learn about cultural and linguistic diversity and how it affects your clinical services.

LANGUAGE VARIATIONS

Traditionally, whether a child has a language disorder is determined on the basis of **norms**, which are the typical behaviors of a reference group of persons. A child whose language performance falls below the norms is said to have a language disorder.

But the idea that there are norms of language use does not mean that English or any language is spoken in one and only one way. No language is spoken in the same way, although variations in spoken language have diminished in this age of electronic communication. Also, American English historically has had less variation than British English. Nonetheless, there are significant differences in the way American English is spoken in different parts of the country.

Variations of a language are called **dialects**. Dialects are different ways of speaking the same language.

Some dialects are based on **geographic regions**; they were originally created by relative isolation of people living in different parts of a country. American English has the following dialects based on geographic regions:

• Central Midland

• Southern

• Southwest

• Northwest

UNIT NOTES

CLASS NOTES

- Northcentral

- Appalachian

- Middle Atlantic

- West Pennsylvania

- New York City

- Eastern New England

Other dialects are based primarily on ethnocultural variables and secondarily on geographic variables. A well-known variety of American English in this category is **Black English Vernacular (BEV)**. Speech-language pathologists serving African-American children should have a good understanding of BEV and its cultural heritage (Dillard, 1972). It is important to remember that:

- BEV is not a degenerate form of some standard English.

- BEV has its variations, too. All of its variations have their own rules, logic, and patterns.

- Not all African-Americans speak BEV.

- Some white people, especially those in southern rural areas, speak elements of BEV.

Still other dialects are due to a speaker's **bilingual status**. In these speakers, the dialect of a second language is influenced by their primary language. For instance, there are **dialects of American English that are based on a primary language**. These are the dialects of the American English spoken by people whose native language is other than English. Thus, we have dialects that are influenced by Spanish, French, Russian, Yiddish, German, Italian, Chinese, Japanese, Punjabi, Hindi, Kannada, and other languages.

Other dialects are due to **individual differences** because each person speaks his or her language in a unique way. A dialect due to individual uniqueness is called an **idiolect**.

Some dialects may be based on a certain **group membership**. Many teenage people, for example, have their own dialects, which may be called **teen-lects**. Similarly, people belonging to different socioeconomic classes may speak different dialects.

Some speakers can speak more than one dialect of their language. Speakers who speak multiple dialects switch from one to the other depending on their conversational partners or audience. This is called **code switching**.

Often, what is considered a standard dialect in a society is simply the variation of a language spoken by the **rich**, the **educated**, and the politically and economically **powerful**. This is why the notion of a standard form of language is prejudicial. The issue is not entirely ethnic.

Consider Professor Henry Higgins's contemptuous judgment of Eliza Doolittle's dialect of the lower social class (*My Fair Lady* by Lerner & Loewe, 1956, p. 109):

> *Look at her—a pris'ner of the gutters;*
> *Condemned by ev'ry syllable she utters.*
> *By right she should be taken out and hung*
> *For the cold blooded murder of the English tongue!*

People, including those in various professions, education, and business often make negative judgments about the intelligence or other kinds of abilities of a person based on how that person speaks. As human service professionals, speech-language pathologists have a special obligation to design appropriate, culturally based, and nondiscriminatory services to all who need them.

LANGUAGE DIFFERENCES VERSUS DISORDERS

Because the issue of language differences has important implications for the profession of speech-language pathology, the American Speech-Language-Hearing Association (ASHA) has taken an official position on it. The Association has stated that "It is the position of the American Speech-Language-Hearing Association that no dialectal variety of English is a disorder or a pathological form of speech or language" (Social dialects position paper, Asha, 1983, p. 45).

All variations or dialects of a language are products of historical, cultural, geographic, social, economic, ethnic, and political factors. No variation is inherently superior to other variations because each variation has its cultural roots. Therefore, no child or client is diagnosed to have a language disorder solely because of a dialectal variation.

Language disorders are found in individuals regardless of the dialects spoken. To determine whether a speaker has a language disorder or simply speaks a different dialect, the speech-language pathologist should know the dialectal variations of English, including BEV and English influenced by a speaker's primary language.

To fully understand the clients you serve, you need to study cultural and linguistic differences. Much has been written about linguistic differences between Standard American English on the one hand and BEV and Spanish-influenced English on the other. Some of these differences are summarized in Reed (1994).

Children of Asian background pose a much greater challenge than any other cultural group because of their extraordinary linguistic diversity. You should consult various sources that are now available on understanding and serving different ethnic groups (Battle, 1993; Cheng, 1991, 1995; Hegde & Davis, 1995; Langdon & Cheng, 1992; Mattes & Omark, 1991; Screen & Anderson, 1994).

ASHA also has recognized that a speaker of a dialect may wish to acquire another dialect and thus seek the services of a speech-language pathologist. The clinician may offer such elective treatment.

Other guidelines in working with children with multicultural background are summarized in the next section.

BILINGUAL AND MULTICULTURAL CHILDREN

Most countries of the world are bilingual and multicultural. The United States is no exception, and it is becoming increasingly so. However, most native English speakers in the United States are unilingual.

A person who is **unilingual** knows only one language.

A person who is **bilingual** knows two languages. Many but not all persons who are bilingual tend to have diverse cultural backgrounds.

A person who is **multilingual** or is a **polyglot** knows more than two languages.

Multilingual and multicultural populations in the United States pose special educational and professional challenges.

More than 18% of the U.S. population speaks a language other than English at home. This means that 42 million Americans are bilingual; some of them are multilingual.

Nearly half of this population does not speak English well. Some do not speak English at all.

Nearly 7 million children with no or limited English proficiency are enrolled in the U.S. public schools. Most of these children are not being served well by the schools.

Contrary to earlier beliefs, bilingualism is not necessarily detrimental to a child's language or academic performance.

Guidelines on Serving Bilingual and Multicultural Children

For the speech-language pathologist, children who are bilingual-multicultural pose special challenges. The clinician should know the general guidelines of

UNIT NOTES

serving children with diverse linguistic and ethnic backgrounds (Hegde & Davis, 1995). In serving such children, the clinician should:

- have a knowledge of both the culture and language of children who are bilingual-multicultural.

- understand the language structure and how the language is used in the client's culture.

- understand how a disorder of communication is evaluated and managed in the culture.

- be knowledgeable in multicultural service delivery issues (how a cultural group reacts to treatment, questions of payment, attendance at treatment sessions, family involvement, and so forth).

- use culturally sensitive, nondiscriminatory assessment tools and treatment materials.

- not think that teaching a second language—be it English or any other language—is her or his duty. That is the duty of the language teacher.

- decide whether a child who is bilingual has a disorder of communication in the primary language, in the second language, or both using culturally and linguistically appropriate assessment methods.

- offer clinical services only when the child has a disorder of communication in either the first language, the second language, or both. To make such a determination, the clinician must understand the child's first language, its rules, and uses.

- refer the child to bilingual clinicians when he or she cannot adequately serve them.

- use the services of an interpreter in assessing the child if bilingual clinicians are not available.

- refer the child to a bilingual clinician if the assessment results document a disorder in the bilingual child's primary language.

- offer services in English if the child is reasonably proficient in English and exhibits disorder in it, and it is in the best interest of the child to offer services in English.

- act as the child's advocate and do everything possible to obtain the needed services for the child.

Instructor's Views and Critical Comments on Language of Children of Diverse Cultural and Linguistic Background

_____

_____

_____

_____

_____

_____

_____

_____

_____

_____

_____

_____

_____

_____

_____

_____

_____

_____

_____

_____

_____

_____

_____

REFERENCES AND READING ASSIGNMENTS

American Speech-Language-Hearing Association. (1983). Social dialects. *Asha, 27,* 23–24.

Read this article to fully understand ASHA's position on social dialects and clinical services.

Battle, D. E. (1993). *Communication disorders in multicultural populations.* Stoneham, MA: Andover Medical Publishers.

Read this book to understand the full scope of multicultural issues in speech-language pathology.

Dillard, J. L. (1972). *Black English.* New York: Random House.

Read this book to understand the cultural heritage and linguistic diversity of Black English.

Cheng, L. L. (1991). *Assessing Asian language performance* (2nd ed.). Oceanside, CA: Academic Communication Associates.

Cheng, L. L. (Ed.). (1995). *Integrating language and learning for inclusion: An Asian-Pacific focus.* San Diego: Singular Publishing Group.

Read these two books by Cheng to find out about Asians and Pacific Islanders, their children, their language background, and assessment and treatment issues.

Hegde, M. N., & Davis, D. (1995). *Clinical methods and practicum in speech-language pathology* (2nd ed.). San Diego: Singular Publishing Group.

Read Chapter 6 on multicultural issues in clinical practicum.

Langdon, H. W., & Cheng, L. L. (Eds.). (1992) *Hispanic children and adults with communication disorders: Assessment and intervention.* Gaithersburg, MD: Aspen Publishers.

Read this book to understand assessment and intervention issues in serving Hispanic children.

Lerner, A., & Loewe, F. (1956). *My fair lady.* New York: Chappel.

Read this delightful play on pride and prejudice associated with dialects as well as gender.

Mattes, L., & Omark, D. (1991). *Speech and language assessment for the bilingually handicapped* (2nd ed.). Oceanside, CA: Academic Communication Associates.

Read this book to find out more about assessment procedures to be used with bilingual children.

Reed, V. (1994). *An introduction to children with language disorders* (2nd ed.). New York: Macmillan Publishing Company.

Read Chapter 10 to understand clinical service delivery issues relative to bilingual-bicultural children.

Screen R. M., & Anderson, N. B. (1994). *Multicultural perspectives in communication disorders.* San Diego: Singular Publishing Group.

Special Assignments From the Instructor:

_____

_____

_____

_____

_____

_____

_____

_____

_____

_____

_____

_____

_____

_____

_____

_____

_____

_____

_____

_____

_____

_____

_____

STUDY QUESTIONS

1. What is a dialect?

   _____

   _____

2. List the major American English dialects:

   _____   _____

   _____   _____

   _____   _____

   _____   _____

   _____

3. What is Black English Vernacular (BEV)? What are some of its distinguishing grammatic features as described in assigned readings?

   _____

   _____

   _____

   _____

   _____

   _____

   _____

   _____

   _____

   _____

   _____

4. What are some of the phonologic features of BEV as described in assigned readings?

   _____

   _____

   _____

   _____

_____

_____

5. Justify the statement that Black English is not a degenerate form of standard or other forms of English:

_____

_____

_____

_____

_____

6. Define the following terms:

Idiolect

_____

_____

Teenlect

_____

_____

Code switching

_____

_____

7. Distinguish between language differences and language disorders:

_____

_____

_____

_____

_____

8. Summarize precisely the ASHA's position on social dialects::

_____

_____

_____

_____

_____

_____

_____

_____

9. Define the following terms:

Unilingual

_____

_____

Bilingual

_____

_____

Multilingual

_____

_____

Polyglot

_____

_____

10. Do speech-language pathologists teach a second language to a child? Why or why not?

_____

_____

_____

_____

11. When can a monolingual English-speaking speech-language pathologist offer direct treatment services to a bilingual child?

_____

_____

_____

_____

12. When can a speech-language pathologist treat a dialectal variation?

_____

_____

_____

_____

13. Why should the clinician understand the language and use of a bilingual child's primary language?

_____

_____

_____

_____

14. What kinds of assessment and treatment tools would you select for multicultural children?

_____

_____

_____

_____

15. As a monolingual, English-speaking clinician, what do you do when you cannot serve a bilingual child who needs speech-language services?

_____

_____

_____

_____

Assessment of Language Disorders

....

- Objectives of Assessment

- Procedures of Assessment

- Measurement Issues in Assessment

- Some Suggestions on Observation and Measurement

- References and Reading Assignments

- Study Questions

....

So far, you have learned about language disorders in a variety of populations. In this Unit, you will learn about language assessment to be completed before starting treatment.

OBJECTIVES OF ASSESSMENT

Before starting treatment, you assess your clients to describe, measure, and understand:

- the communication problem (or the presenting complaint) as the family or clients see it

- the beginning and the course of the problem as the family understands it

- how the family has handled the problem

- any previous assessment and treatment the client may have received

- the outcome of previous clinical services and the reasons for the present attempt to seek services

- the family history, constellation, expectations, and support for intervention

- the child's communication and physical development

- the current communication and related skills of the child with an emphasis on the presenting problem (such as language delay or disorder)

- the desired skills that are lacking or produced at low frequency

- the associated clinical conditions (such as hearing impairment, motor deficits, or mental retardation)

- the strengths and limitations of the child and his or her family

- the communicative, social, and educational demands made on the client

- when possible, potential instigating and maintaining causes of the language disorder (diagnosis)

- to the extent possible, an initial treatment program

- the potential outcome of the suggested treatment plan (prognosis)

See Reed (1994), Weiss, Tomblin, and Robin (1994), Paul (1995), and Nelson (1993) for different views on the objectives of assessment.

PROCEDURES OF ASSESSMENT

The objectives of assessment are achieved through:

1. Case History: You take a case history to find out about the child, his or her communicative problems, the family, health of the child, home environment, educational background of the child, previous assessment or treatment; results of such previous procedures, and so forth. If available, you can obtain reports from clinicians who have served the child.

2. Interview: After obtaining the case history, you interview the parents, the client, or both. The purpose of the interview is to obtain more information, and clarification of information provided on the case history form. More information may be sought on the child's speech and language development, how the family interacts with the child, what educational goals are being set, the problems in realizing those goals, the child's social development, and other related issues.

3. Orofacial Examination: You make an orofacial examination of the speech structures of the face and mouth to assess whether there are gross anatomic and physiologic deviations that could cause the speech or language disorder. You observe the tongue mobility, movements of the lips and the soft palate, and the overall structural integrity of the oral-facial complex. Such obvious factors as facial paralysis and cleft palate may be noted during this examination.

4. Hearing Screening: All children and adults who are assessed for a disorder of communication must be given a hearing screening test. This is done to rule out the presence of hearing loss; if the client fails the hearing screening, a referral is made to an audiologist for a complete audiological evaluation.

5. Language Sampling: Recording an adequate language sample is the most important step in language assessment. You should take the following steps in obtaining a language sample from a child:

- Audio record the language sample.

- Observe and record the pattern of interaction between the child and the mother.

- Engage the child in conversational speech on a separate occasion.

- Include siblings if accompanied to the clinic; let them talk to each other as you observe.

- Do not rush the child; let the child get used to the clinical situation.

- Use toys, pictures, and objects and let the child talk about them. Select the stimulus materials that are appropriate for the child's family, linguistic, and cultural background.

- Do not talk too much; let the child do most of the talking.

- Ask open-ended questions. Do not ask too many questions that evoke *yes* or *no* answers (e. g., ask "Who is this?" instead of "Is this Mickey?"; "What do you do Saturday mornings?" instead of "Do you watch cartoons on Saturday mornings?").

- See if toys and pictures limit verbal interactions; some children can get lost in play activities; there-fore, as soon as possible, move on to conversational speech about topics the child can talk about.

- Ask various questions about the child's life, school, activities, favorite TV shows, friends, birthday parties, vacation, and so forth.

- Tell a story and ask the child to retell it.

- Vary the activities and stimulus materials.

- Take notes on the context of utterances, as without such notes, some utterances may be meaningless on the audio tape.

- Obtain a second language sample if the first did not produce an adequate sample of language skills of the child.

Collect a sample of **50 to 100 utterances**. Expect to spend about **30 minutes** to collect an adequate sample, but remember the duration depends on the individual child.

6. Administration of Standardized Tests: Most clinicians administer selected standardized tests of language development and production. It is believed that standardized tests, as long as they are valid and reliable, provide the best and the most practical information about the language abilities of the child. The child's performance is then compared against the norms provided by the test author. If the child's performance falls below the norm specified for the child's age level, then a language delay or disorder is diagnosed.

Select tests that are reliable, valid, comprehensive, and culturally and linguistically appropriate. See the next section for limitations of standardized tests.

7. Initial Analysis of Results and Recommendations: At the end of the assessment session, the clinician makes an initial analysis of results to gain an overall impression of the child. The clinician then interviews the client, the parent, or both to make tentative clinical recommendations based on the assessment results.

8. Final Analysis and Report Writing: The clinician finally makes a more complete analysis of assessment results after the assessment session. The clinician listens to the conversational speech samples, examines the notes and observations made during the assessment, and considers any reports received from other professionals to analyze various aspects of communication, including:

- the kinds of words used, and if relevant and practical, an estimated size of the vocabulary

- the mean length of utterance

- the length of typical (mode) utterance

- the shortest and the longest utterance

- the grammatic morphemes that the child produces and those that the child does not produce

- the syntactic structures the child produces and those that the child does not produce

- the types and varieties of sentence structures the child uses

- pragmatic skills including eye contact, turn taking, topic maintenance, conversational repair, and so forth

- comprehension of spoken language

- phonological skills and the presence of articulation or phonological problems

- voice quality and the presence of any voice disorders

- fluency and the presence of fluency disorders

The clinician may use one of the several **computer software programs** to analyze language samples. These include Lingquest 1 (Mordecai & Palin, 1982); Systematic Analysis of Language Transcripts (SALT; Miller & Chapman, 1983); and Computerized

Profiling (Long & Fey, 1993). See Reed (1994) for a brief description and evaluation of these programs.

Eventually, the clinician writes a formal report in which she or he makes the final recommendations and suggests a treatment plan.

See Weiss, Tomblin, and Robin (1994), Reed (1994), Nelson (1993), Paul (1995), and Lund and Duchan (1988) to better understand the range of procedures used in assessing language disorders in children.

MEASUREMENT ISSUES IN ASSESSMENT

In its technical and essential aspects, assessment is the reliable measurement of specified language behaviors under varied stimulus conditions and in different response modes. Therefore, the clinician should be aware of certain measurement issues that are linked to assessment:

Reliability of Measurement: Because a single language sample does not demonstrate reliability, the clinician needs to obtain additional samples. This may be done when the client returns for the first treatment session. Brief language samples should be recorded during the first two or three treatment sessions.

Reliability and Validity of Standardized Tests: Standardized tests may or may not have acceptable levels of reliability. Even if they do, the normatively reported reliability does not demonstrate the reliability of measures obtained on a specific child. Therefore, the burden of reliability rests on repeated conversational speech samples.

Subject Sampling in the Standardization Process: All standardized tests sample subjects, and there are few or no tests that sample all segments of the population. Therefore, many tests are not applicable across population groups. This is especially true of culturally diverse populations because of their underrepresentation in the normative samples.

Response Sampling in the Standardization Process: Standardized tests, even when they sample subjects adequately, tend to sample behaviors inadequately. That is, a behavior tested, such as a regular plural, is tested in only one or two contexts. This is inadequate behavior sampling, a factor to which test developers pay little attention.

Follow these guidelines in using standardized tests:

- Do not select a test whose reliability is unknown or unacceptable.

- Do not use a test whose normative sample does not include subjects who represent your client; consider all relevant variables: socioeconomic class, urban-rural populations, and cultural, linguistic, and ethnic background.

- Do not use a test as the sole measure to make clinical judgments.

- Do not supplement a test result with that of another test; supplement it with language samples. Remember that from a measurement standpoint, varied and multiple measures do not mean multiple tests.

- Follow the test developers' procedures in administration of tests and interpretation of results.

- Practice test administration before you use it on a client.

- Always be prepared to use alternative procedures; most importantly, client-specific measures.

Client-Specific Measures: In most cases, client-specific measures are preferable to standardized tests. Client-specific procedures form a valid basis for developing client-specific treatment. A detailed conversational speech sample, additional brief samples recorded subsequently, and supplemented by home speech samples provide useful, client-specific data. These samples are evoked through client-specific, culturally appropriate stimulus

UNIT NOTES

materials, instead of standard stimuli. The procedures of client-specific measures are more easily adapted to suit culturally diverse clients than are standardized procedures.

Baselines as Extended Measurement: To overcome the reliability problems inherent to traditional assessment procedures, the clinician should establish baselines of communicative behaviors targeted for treatment. **Baselines** are measures of target behaviors in the absence of planned treatment. Because they are extended and repeated, they provide more reliable assessment data than tests and other procedures. However, baselines are established only on behaviors selected for immediate treatment. Based on baseline data, the clinician cannot make statements about overall communicative performance of a client.

Baseline procedures will be described in the next unit.

SOME SUGGESTIONS ON OBSERVATION AND MEASUREMENT

The assessment procedures you use with a given child will depend upon the verbal repertoire of the child. For example, a child who is nonverbal is assessed differently than a child who is highly verbal with only a few grammatic or pragmatic problems. Therefore, the clinician needs to have a rough idea about the verbal level of the child even before selecting the assessment procedures. Information obtained through case history and interview will help to gain an initial impression of child's general language level.

Besides the previously described case history and interview, the clinician should informally observe the child and the accompanying family members to better understand the verbal level of the child. The clinician should take note of the following:

- How do the child and the mother interact? Do they gesture to each other?

UNIT NOTES

- Does the child use words, phrases, sentences? Does the child seem to understand sentences or only words?

- How does the child interact with you, the clinician? Spontaneously verbal? Answered questions? Told you his or her name? Willing to talk?

- Shy and withdrawn? Hiding behind the mother?

- What does the case history suggest? A nonverbal child? Minimally verbal (words and gestures only)?

Informal observations of this kind will help you determine the approximate verbal level of the child. Generally speaking, the verbal level of a child may vary between nonverbal and essentially normal with only a few advanced language features missing.

The following somewhat arbitrary verbal levels and the procedures specified under them are to be used only as rough and not necessarily comprehensive suggestions for completing the assessment of verbal behaviors of children with language disorders.

1. Nonverbal: The child is essentially speechless. In this case, the clinician should assess:

- Gestures, signs, and symbols the child may be using

- Vocalization or imitation of nonspeech sounds

- Vocalization or imitation of any speech sounds

- Nonverbal responses to verbal stimuli including correct pointing, discriminating between objects (comprehension)

- Imitations of simple words and phrases

- Spontaneous production of words

Even though the indications are that the child is essentially nonverbal, assessment always probes slightly higher levels to make sure. That is why imitation and spontaneous production of selected words are probed.

The assessment of children who are nonverbal poses challenges because of the presence of multiple handicaps requiring assessment by a team of specialists. Most of the procedures used are client-specific.

2. Minimally verbal: This child produces simple, isolated word responses; perhaps a few phrases; but no sentence structure. In this case, the clinician should assess:

- Everything mentioned under Level 1

- Naming common objects, toys, family members, items of clothing and food

- Counting simple numbers, reciting the days of the week

- Word combinations; production and imitation of simple phrases

- Production or comprehension of certain grammatic morphemes such as the present progressive *ing* and the plural morphemes

- Production and comprehension of simple sentence structures

3. Word combinations and some connected speech. The child at this level may on occasion produce simple sentence forms. In this case, the clinician should assess:

- Everything mentioned under Levels 1 and 2

- Answers to simple questions

- Simple conversational speech samples

- Assessment of various grammatic features, syntactic structures, sentence types

- The mean length of responses, the length of typical responses, and so forth

• comprehension of conversational speech

Assessment of a child who produces some connected speech places a greater emphasis on language samples. Those who wish to administer standardized tests will find many opportunities to do so.

4. Apparently normal language, deficiencies in advanced aspects of language: You will see children whose language problems are subtle. The child may have near-normal language performance but a few advanced language concepts or structures may not be used or may be misused (e.g., does not understand the difference between *ask* and *tell*; lack of passive, compound, or complex sentence forms). In such cases:

• assess mostly through conversational speech

• use client-specific procedures to sample the particular behaviors of interest

Remember, the described levels are arbitrary. Children do not neatly fall into one of the levels. The levels illustrate a range of verbal behaviors.

Instructor's Views and Critical Comments on Assessing Language Disorders in Children

_____

_____

_____

_____

_____

_____

_____

_____

_____

_____

_____

_____

_____

_____

_____

_____

_____

_____

_____

_____

_____

_____

REFERENCES AND READING ASSIGNMENTS

Long, S., & Fey, M. (1993). Computerized Profiling (Macintosh version 1.0, MS-DOS version 7.1) [Computer software]. San Antonio, TX: Psychological Corporation.

Consider using this computerized program to assess language.

Lund, N. J., & Duchan, J. F. (1988). *Assessing children's language in naturalistic contexts*. Englewood, NJ: Prentice-Hall.

Read this book to understand assessment in naturalistic contexts.

Miller, J., & Chapman, R. (1983). SALT: Systematic analysis of language transcripts [Computer software]. Madison: Language Analysis Laboratory, Weisman Center, University of Wisconsin.

Consider using this computerized program to assess language.

Mordecai, D., & Palin, M. (1982). Lingquest 1 & 2 [Computer software]. Napa, CA: Lingquest Software.

Consider using this computerized program to assess language.

Nelson, N. W. (1993). *Childhood language disorders in context*. New York: Macmillan.

Read Chapter 6 on assessment of language disorders in children.

Paul, R. (1995). *Language disorders from infancy through adolescence*. St. Louis: Mosby.

Read sections on assessment in Chapters 7, 8, 9, 12, and 14.

Reed, V. (1994). *An introduction to children with language disorders* (2nd ed.). New York: Macmillan Publishing Company.

Read Chapter 14 on assessment and diagnosis of language disorders in children.

Weis, A. L., Tomblin, J. B., & Robin, D. A. (1994). Language disorders. In J. B. Tomblin, H. L. Morris, & D. C. Spreistersbach (Eds.), *Diagnosis in speech-language pathology* (pp. 99–134). San Diego: Singular Publishing Group.

Use this book as one of your resources on assessment and diagnosis in speech-language pathology.

Special Assignments From the Instructor:

_____

_____

_____

_____

_____

_____

_____

_____

_____

_____

_____

_____

_____

_____

_____

_____

_____

_____

_____

_____

_____

_____

_____

_____

_____

_____

STUDY QUESTIONS

1. Describe briefly the objectives of assessment:

   _____

   _____

   _____

   _____

   _____

   _____

   _____

   _____

2. Describe the areas of information a case history concentrates on:

   _____

   _____

   _____

   _____

   _____

   _____

   _____

3. Why do you interview the parents or clients?

   _____

   _____

   _____

   _____

   _____

   _____

4. Why do you do an orofacial examination?

   _____

   _____

   _____

   _____

_____

_____

5. Describe some of the pragmatic skills that should be assessed:

_____

_____

_____

_____

_____

6. Describe how a language sample should be recorded:

_____

_____

_____

_____

_____

7. Describe how you would analyze the language samples and other assessment data:

_____

_____

_____

_____

_____

_____

_____

8. What are reliability and validity of standardized tests?

_____

_____

_____

9. What are the limitations of standardized tests?

10. What are client-specific procedures? Give an example:

11. What are baselines? Why do you need them?

12. How do you initially determine the verbal level of a child?

_____

_____

13. What would you concentrate on in assessing a child who is nonverbal?

_____

_____

_____

_____

_____

_____

14. What language skills would you assess in a child who uses word combinations and connected speech?

_____

_____

_____

_____

_____

15. What is the primary method of assessing advanced language skills?

_____

_____

_____

_____

_____

UNIT 10

Language Treatment: Basic Procedures

. . . .

- Steps in Developing a Language Treatment Program

- Selection of Target Behaviors

- Planning a Sequence of Treatment

- Selection of Stimulus Materials

- Establishing Baselines

- Writing a Treatment and Maintenance Plan

- Implementing the Treatment Plan

- A Note on Comprehension Training

- A Note on the Degree of Structure of Training Sessions

- References and Reading Assignments

- Study Questions

. . . .

This Unit and the next three Units are about treatment of language disorders. In this Unit, you will learn a basic language treatment procedure. In Unit 11, you will learn about some variations and additional procedures. In Unit 12 you will learn about teaching conversational skills. In Unit 13, the final unit, you will learn about maintenance procedures.

STEPS IN DEVELOPING A LANGUAGE TREATMENT PROGRAM

The basic treatment procedure includes the following steps:

1. Selection of target behaviors

2. Planning a sequence of treatment

3. Selection of stimulus materials

4. Establishing baselines

5. Writing a treatment and maintenance plan

6. Implementing the treatment plan

7. Implementing the maintenance plan

Six of these 7 steps will be described in this unit. The last step is described in Unit 13.

SELECTION OF TARGET BEHAVIORS

The first step is to select target behaviors that are appropriate for the child. Independent groups of teachable target behaviors are called **functional response classes**. Teaching some of the responses within a class is sufficient for the child to produce all of them. For instance, nouns that take the plural *s* morpheme may form a class. It is not necessary to teach every word that takes that plural morpheme. Teaching a few exemplars is sufficient.

UNIT NOTES

Functional response classes may be words, phrases, sentence forms; morphologic features; syntactic structures (selected types of sentences); pragmatic features; or cognitive skills.

Target response classes selected for training:

- should be client-specific (appropriate to the given child)

- should be useful to the child

- should enhance the child's communicative skills in natural settings

- should help build more complex skills

- should help the child meet his or her social and educational demands

PLANNING A SEQUENCE OF TREATMENT

Most children who need language services need to learn multiple target behaviors because these children are deficient in many aspects of language. However, not all behaviors can be simultaneously taught. Therefore, the target behaviors must be sequenced.

In sequencing the language targets, many clinicians use the normative approach: teach the behaviors according to their normal sequence of acquisition. There is no compelling clinical evidence that dictates the use of normative sequence.

Others sequence targets on a client-specific basis. They are willing to experiment and find out which sequence works the best for a given child.

Most skills have their own sequence: you need to teach certain language skills before certain other skills can be taught or be meaningful to teach. For example, the child needs to learn the main verbs before the child can learn the present progressive *ing*; nouns before plural inflections, and so forth.

CLASS NOTES

Generally, clinicians move from:

- more basic structures to progressively more advanced structures (words, phrases, sentences)

- simpler to more complex skills

- structured, evoked responses to more spontaneous, naturally occurring responses

- controlled utterances to conversational speech

- language produced in the clinic to that produced in natural settings

- clinician-evoked language to language evoked by significant people in the child's life

SELECTION OF STIMULUS MATERIALS

After selecting the target behaviors, you select s timulus materials needed to teach them. The stimuli may be books, pictures, objects (including toys), and events you act out. The selected stimulus material should be:

- colorful and attractive to the child

- realistic

- unambiguous so they are effective in evoking target responses

- culturally and ethnically appropriate

Preferably, select objects from the child's environment. Ask parents to bring the child's toys. Create your own collection of stimulus materials.

ESTABLISHING BASELINES

Before starting treatment, you must establish baselines (or baserates) on behaviors that will be trained immediately. You do not baserate all the missing language responses; you baserate only those that will be taught soon.

Baselines are response rates in the absence of the planned intervention. Baselines help:

- establish the need for treatment

- document improvement in the child's language under treatment

- modify treatment procedure if there is no improvement

- establish clinician accountability

Baseline Procedures

Write target behavior exemplars. To baserate a target behavior, you need to write exemplars of that behavior. For instance, if the present progressive *ing* is a treatment target, you need a word (walk*ing*), a phrase (he walk*ing*), or a sentence (he is walk*ing*) in which it is used. Each word, phrase, or sentence that contains the target feature is an **exemplar**. Prepare 15 to 20 exemplars for each target behavior. Whether your exemplars are words, phrases, or sentences depend on the child and the level of training.

Select the stimulus materials. Select pictures or objects to represent each of the exemplars from your collection of stimulus materials.

Baserate the responses. To accurately calculate the percent correct response rates, use the discrete trial procedure. A **discrete trial procedure** is the one in which each stimulus presentation is a separate and discrete opportunity for the client to produce the target response. For instance, in baserating the evoked production of plural morpheme *s*, take the following steps:

1. Place the picture of two cups in front of the child.

2. Ask the child "Timmy, what do you see?"

3. Give the child 3 to 5 seconds to respond.

4. Record the child's response on a recording sheet.

5. Take away the picture.

6. Wait for about 3 seconds.

Start the next trial (it may be a different exemplar: *Two books*) as with Step 1.

If you have 20 exemplars, administer each once without modeling and once with modeling. On a modeled trial, ask the question and immediately model the correct response.

Calculate the percent correct response rate. For instance, you may find that a child's production of the plural *s* morpheme is 5%.

Baserate and calculate the percent correct response rate for all targets that will be taught immediately. Do not baserate language skills that will be taught later as dated baserates are not valid. All target skills should be baserated just before they are taught.

The discrete trial baserates must be supplemented with a **conversational speech sample** designed to evoke the baserated target behaviors. This would probably be the second sample; the first one would have been obtained in the assessment process.

WRITING A TREATMENT AND MAINTENANCE PLAN

It is better to write a detailed treatment plan before you start treatment. In some cases, a few initial sessions of treatment need to be conducted before finalizing the treatment procedures. In any case, you should begin the process of planning the entire treatment sequence, treatment and probe procedures, and the maintenance program. You may finalize the treatment plan after a few sessions of treatment.

IMPLEMENTING THE TREATMENT PLAN

A behavioral definition of treatment is that it is the **management of a behavioral contingency between stimulus events, response topographies, and response consequences**. A picture, an object, or an event you create is a stimulus event. The child's target response to this stimulus event specifies response topography. (Topography refers to the form or shape of the response; a word and a phrase have different topographies.) What the clinician does when the child gives a correct response or does not give a correct response is the contingent consequence. A contingent consequence is the one that follows a behavior immediately.

An overall contingency is an abstract relation between stimuli, responses, and consequences. This is what you manage in treatment.

It is likely that with many children with language problems, the initial sessions will be more structured than later sessions. Children who are minimally verbal, mentally retarded, autistic, and those who exhibit limited attentional skills benefit a great deal by structured treatment sessions.

As the child masters the initial skills, and as the treatment progresses to more complex skill levels, you gradually reduce the structure of sessions and eventually arrange treatment sessions that resemble more naturalistic communicative situations.

Your initial, structured training trials also will use the discrete trial procedure. Because in most cases you should model the correct response, the following illustrates a modeled discrete training trial:

1. Place the stimulus picture or object in front of the child; act out an event or demonstrate an action that will serve as the stimulus.

2. Ask the evoking question and model the correct response immediately (e. g., "Timmy, what do you see, Say *I see two books*").

3. Give the child a few seconds to respond.

4. If the child correctly imitates the response, praise the child and reinforce in other ways.

5. If the response is incorrect, give corrective feedback. For example, say "No" or "That is not right."

6. Record the response on the recording sheet.

7. Remove the picture or object for a few seconds to show that a trial has ended.

Start the next trial after the brief pause.

Present the same stimulus unless the errors persist; in which case, present a new stimulus item. When the child begins to imitate the response, do not lose it by shifting to a new stimulus.

From this point on, you will have to make a series of clinical decisions as to when to stop modeling, when is an exemplar learned, when to probe, when to move on to another target behavior, and so forth. Criteria for making such decisions are described in the next section.

Criteria For Clinical Decisions

What follows is a series of suggested criteria that help make clinical decisions. Clinicians use more or less rigid criteria. You may have good reasons to change them; be consistent with your stated criteria.

Criterion to stop modeling

Stop modeling when the client gives five consecutively correct imitated responses. Introduce evoked trials which do not include modeling.

On an evoked trial, present the stimulus, ask the question, and wait for a few seconds; if the response is correct, reinforce it, and if it is not correct, give corrective feedback.

Criterion to reinstate modeling

Reinstate the modeled trials if the client gives incorrect responses on two consecutive evoked trials.

Use this criterion during the first stage of evoked trials; later, be more liberal: perhaps four or five consecutively wrong responses on evoked trials may be noted before reinstating modeling.

When correct responses on the evoked trials become more consistent, you should make a decision as to whether the client has learned the first exemplar.

Exemplar training criterion

When the client gives 10 consecutively correct responses on evoked trials, move on to the next exemplar.

This is the **exemplar training criterion**. Note that this criterion only says that a given exemplar, not the feature, is learned. That is, when a child meets the training criterion on such an exemplar as *the boy is running*, it only means that that specific utterance is learned; the feature of present progressive is not mastered yet.

Teach four to six exemplars to this exemplar training criterion before you conduct the first probe to see if the client can produce the language structure in some new (untrained contexts). That is, to determine that the client has tentatively learned the feature or behavior (such as the plural morpheme or the possessive or the present progressive) use the following probe criterion; note that although the exemplar criterion states that a particular exemplar of a target behavior is trained, the probe criterion states that the entire feature or behavior is tentatively trained.

Probe Criterion

The probe criterion is a 90% correct probe response rate on a particular language structure or behavior.

When the client meets the probe criterion on one feature, structure, or behavior, you move on to the next feature, structure, or behavior. In each case, then, you move on to another target feature or behavior when the client meets the probe criterion.

If the client does not meet the probe criterion (less than 90% correct probe response rate), give training on additional exemplars. Use the untrained items to provide more training. After having trained two to four more items to the training criterion, probe again. Probes, therefore, determine whether you begin training on a new target behavior or give training on additional exemplars of the same behavior.

The Probe Procedure

A **probe** is a procedure designed to assess the initial generalization of a target response to selected untrained stimuli. Probes help assess the production of newly taught behaviors in new contexts.

There are two kinds of probes: intermixed and pure. On **intermixed probes**, both trained and untrained stimulus items are presented. On **pure probes**, only the untrained items are presented. Responses to untrained items are not reinforced whereas those to trained items are reinforced if correct.

In the beginning stages of training, only intermixed probes are used. Pure probes are reserved for later stages of training.

Use the following schedule for an intermixed probe:

Stimulus Items	Responses
1. Trained item	
2. Untrained item	
3. Trained item	
4. Untrained item	

Re-use the trained items. Use at least 10 untrained items. These will be the same as the baserated items.

Calculate the percent correct response rate based only on the responses to the probe items. Ignore the responses to the trained items. Alternate training and probe until the probe criterion is met for a given behavior. Begin training on the next behavior. With this procedure, complete training on all the selected target skills or features.

In the next unit, you will learn about training the target behaviors at more complex levels and to use additional procedures. Variations in treatment procedures also will be presented in the next unit.

A NOTE ON COMPREHENSION TRAINING

A child who does not produce some aspect of language also may not understand it. The child who cannot say "shut the door" may not understand when someone else says it. The child, in this case, lacks comprehension as well as production.

Soon after selecting some target behaviors, you may decide on training comprehension. For example, after having selected the prepositions *on* and *in* for training, you ask the child to "show me the cat is on the chair," "show me the cat is in the box"; and so on, until the child gives a certain number of correct pointing responses. In the comprehension training, the client is not asked to produce the target verbal response. In most cases, the client gives a nonverbal response (correct pointing, for instance).

UNIT NOTES

There is some evidence to suggest that comprehension training may induce comprehension, but not production. However, when you train production, comprehension is typically induced. Though more research is needed, an economical strategy is to first train production and then probe for comprehension. If comprehension still is lacking, it should be trained. In most cases, this training may be unnecessary if production is trained first.

A NOTE ON THE DEGREE OF STRUCTURE OF TRAINING SESSIONS

Some clinicians advocate highly structured sessions whereas others suggest loose structure. Each has its advantages and disadvantages. Tight structure is good for certain clients and is generally more efficient in establishing target behaviors especially at basic topographic levels. But tight structure is weak in promoting generalization and maintenance, and in teaching conversational speech. Loose structure is better at these. However, loose structure is less efficient in establishing behaviors and may not be suitable to certain clients (e.g., clients who are distractible or mentally retarded who need massed training trials).

The degree of structure is a matter of client specificity, not a matter of clinician's preference. Those who need a tight structure should get it and those who do well with loose structure should not be subjected to tight structure.

Even when tight structure is needed, it is needed only in the early stages of training. In subsequent stages, loose structure that permits a more naturalistic communication context for training should be used. Thus, in all cases, regardless of the degree of initial structure, latter stages of treatment will use progressively less structure. In the very final stage, in which naturalistic conversation is taught, there is no more structure than what is normal in such interactions.

CLASS NOTES

Instructor's Views and Critical Comments on Language Treatment: Basic Procedures _____

_____

_____

_____

_____

_____

_____

_____

_____

_____

_____

_____

_____

_____

_____

_____

_____

_____

_____

_____

_____

_____

REFERENCES AND READING ASSIGNMENTS

Hegde, M. N., & Gierut, J. (1979). The operant training and generalization of pronouns and a verb form in a language delayed child. *Journal of Communication Disorders, 12,* 23–34

Hegde, M. N., & McConn, J. (1981). Language training: Some data on response classes and generalization to an occupational setting. *Journal of Speech and Hearing Disorders, 46,* 353–358

Hegde, M. N., Noll, M. J., & Pecora, R. (1979). A study of some factors affecting generalization of language training. *Journal of Speech and Hearing Disorders, 44,* 301–320.

Read the three articles to understand procedures and the empirical bases of the treatment procedures described in this unit.

McCormick, L., & Schiefelbusch, R. L. (1990). *Early language intervention.* Columbus, OH: Merrill.

Read this book on intervention techniques used with young children.

Nelson, N. W. (1993). *Childhood language disorders in context.* New York: Merrill.

Read assigned chapters or sections on intervention.

Paul, R. (1995). *Language disorders from infancy through adolescence.* St. Louis: Mosby.

Read sections on treatment in Chapters 7 through 10 for various language treatment techniques.

Reed, V. (1994). *An introduction to children with language disorders* (2nd ed.). New York: Macmillan.

Read Chapter 15 on language intervention

Special Assignments From the Instructor:

_____

_____

_____

_____

_____

_____

_____

_____

_____

_____

_____

_____

_____

_____

_____

_____

_____

_____

_____

_____

_____

_____

_____

STUDY QUESTIONS

1. List the steps involved in developing a basic treatment program:

   _____   _____

   _____   _____

   _____   _____

2. What are functional response classes? Give examples:

   _____

   _____

   _____

   _____

3. List four grammatic morphemes that could serve as target behaviors:

   _____   _____

   _____   _____

4. List four syntactic structures that could serve as target behaviors:

   _____   _____

   _____   _____

5. List four pragmatic features that could serve as target behaviors:

   _____   _____

   _____   _____

6. Describe the characteristics of target responses:

   _____   _____

   _____   _____

   _____   _____

7. Specify the general sequence of training:

   _____   _____

   _____   _____

   _____   _____

   _____   _____

8. List the characteristics of stimulus materials:

_____   _____

_____   _____

9. Define baselines and state why we need them:

_____

_____

_____

_____

10. Specify the steps involved in administering baseline trials:

_____

_____

_____

_____

_____

_____

11. Define treatment:

_____

_____

_____

_____

12. Specify the steps involved in administering a discrete trial training procedure:

_____

_____

_____

_____

_____

_____

_____

13. When do you stop modeling?

_____

_____

_____

_____

14. When do you reinstate modeling?

_____

_____

_____

_____

15. When do you move on to the next exemplar?

_____

_____

_____

_____

16. What is a probe criterion?

_____

_____

_____

_____

17. What is a probe?

_____

_____

_____

_____

18. Distinguish between intermixed and pure probes:

_____

_____

_____

_____

19. Do you reinforce responses given to probe items?

_____

_____

_____

_____

20. What do you do when the client does not meet the probe criterion?

_____

_____

_____

_____

Language Treatment: Variations and Additional Procedures

. . . .

- Complex Levels of Training

- Additional Procedures

- Response Reduction Procedures

- Procedural Modifications

- References and Reading Assignments

- Study Questions

. . . .

UNIT NOTES

In this Unit, you will find descriptions of complex levels of language training, several additional procedures, variations in language treatment procedures, and procedural modifications.

COMPLEX LEVELS OF TRAINING

In most cases, clinicians begin treatment by teaching words, grammatic morphemes in words or phrases, and pragmatic structures at simpler topographic levels. When the child meets the initial and tentative training criterion (a 90% or better probe response rate, as you recall), clinicians move on to more complex levels of training.

Also, clinicians initially select a small number of targets on which they work in every treatment session. For example, a clinician might begin treatment with four grammatic morphemes.

When one or more of the initially selected target behaviors reach the tentative training criterion, the clinician has two options.

Option 1. The clinician may wait until all four or six (or whatever the number) of initially selected behaviors reach the tentative training criterion before moving on to a higher level of training. That is, the training will continue on the same initial level of complexity on the targets that have not met the training criterion.

Option 2. As soon as the client meets the tentative training criterion on a particular behavior, the clinician moves to the next level of training on that behavior. Training will continue on the other initial targets at the initial level of complexity. In this case, different behaviors will be trained at different levels; at a certain point, one behavior may be at the highest level of training (conversational speech), another may be one level below this, a third behavior may be at the second level of complexity, and the fourth behavior may be at the initial level of response complexity.

In language treatment, response complexity is typically graded as follows:

- Words

- Phrases

- Simpler, shorter sentences

- Longer, more complex sentences

- Conversational speech

It is extremely important to move the client to the conversational mode and reinforce the production of behaviors in that mode. A failure to reinforce the target behaviors in the conversational mode may be the reason why many clients do not generalize their newly learned language behaviors to more naturalistic settings. Speech is not typically evoked by pictures on discrete trials; it is evoked by the events of the environment. Therefore, in the final stages of intervention, the clinician should have the client produce the target language skills under natural conditions of communication.

ADDITIONAL PROCEDURES

Clinicians typically use several specific treatment procedures in various stages of training. Some of the following procedures are used in almost all treatment programs (shaping, modeling, instructions, prompting, manual guidance) whereas some of the others are specific training programs to teach advanced language skills (incidental teaching, script therapy, joint book reading).

Shaping

A child who does not imitate a response needs the **shaping procedure** in which successive approximations of the target response is reinforced. For example, if the child cannot imitate the word *Mommy*, you ask the child to make an *mmm* sound or to simply put the lips together, or to move the lips; and out of these initial responses, you shape the terminal response. In gradual steps, you add more complex features of the terminal response. The *mmm* sound is shaped into *Ma*, which is then shaped into *Mom*, which is finally shaped into *Mommy*.

In shaping a response:

- Break a complex or difficult response into smaller, more easily learned components

- Identify an initial response the child can imitate or produce with manual guidance

- Identify intermediate responses that are linked

- Identify the terminal response (the final target)

- Begin training with the initial response

- Use instructions, modeling, manual guidance, and prompting

- Reinforce the imitated or spontaneously produced responses

- As the initial response is reliably produced, move to the next response

- Each time one of the intermediate responses is reliably produced, shift training to include additional components of the terminal response

- End training with the terminal response; provide more training on this

Instructions

Most clients, even young children, can benefit from instructions that describe a target behavior and, when appropriate, specify how it is produced.

- Give instructions in simple, direct language

- Combine them with modeling

- Assess the client's understanding of instructions (e.g., ask the client to repeat the instruction)

- Repeat instructions throughout training as found necessary

Modeling

This may be an indispensable procedure in speech and language training. Modeling displays the target behavior for the client. When combined with instructions and manual guidance, modeling may be very effective. Modeling is used in two ways in language training. In most behavioral training programs, the clinician models and requires the child to imitate the modeled target response. In some linguistically oriented approaches, the clinician goes on modeling target responses without requiring imitation. There is much controlled evidence about the efficacy of modeling followed by imitation. Such evidence is lacking for mere modeling that is not followed by imitation.

Prompting

Many children need prompting soon after the modeling is withdrawn. Gestures sometimes work as prompts and help evoke responses from an unsure child (for example, the gesture of drinking from a cup to evoke the response *drinking*). Instead of completely withdrawing modeling, you can withdraw it partially; partial modeling works as prompts: "Say I see two . . . ," can often evoke the response *books* (when shown pictures). Next, the clinician might say, " Say I see, . . . ;" then, "Timmy, say, I . . ." This method of reducing the power of a stimulus is called **fading**. Every time you use prompting, you also should use fading.

Manual Guidance

This technique involves providing physical assistance to execute a response. It is perhaps more useful in shaping a response and in comprehension training. For example, the clinician might gently push the jaw downward to encourage the child to open the mouth and vocalize. Similarly, the clinician might take the hand of the child and touch the right picture when comprehension is being trained.

Expansion

This is another technique many clinicians use. It is a procedure of expanded modeling: the clinician repeats what the child just said while adding grammatic features the child did not use. Child language research has shown that parents expand children's utterances to make them grammatically more complete. For example, the child says "Mommy coming," looking at the mother coming through the door. The father then may expand the child's utterance by saying, "Mommy *is* coming." In this expanded utterance, the father added the missing auxiliary *is* to the child's utterance. Some clinicians simply go on expanding the child's utterances without expecting the child to imitate the expanded utterance. The effectiveness of such a procedure has not been established. If the clinician asks the child to imitate the expanded utterance and then reinforces the child's response, then expansion may be effective. For example: in a conversational situation, the child says "Jenny hat"; the clinician expands it by saying "Jenny's hat" and asks the child, "Please say "Jenny's hat." The child then imitates "Jenny's hat" and the clinician says "Excellent! That is Jenny's hat."

Extension

In this method, the clinician comments upon the child's utterance to add additional meaning; it also is known as expatiation. While expansions target grammatic features, extensions target semantic features; imitation may or may not be required; if required, it is a more direct language training method; if not, it is an indirect language stimulation procedure.

In using extensions, the clinician arranges a loose training structure with toys, books, and pictures. As the child produces semantically limited, unclear, and ambiguous utterances, the clinician extends them to include more meaning. For instance, the child might say "horsie running"; the clinician then might extend the child's utterances in different ways, including "Yes, the horsie is running fast," and "Sure the horsie is going to win the race" and so forth. We need more experimental research on the effects of extension on the child's language.

Recast

Expansion of a child's utterance type into a different type of utterance is known as **recast**. This technique is used in play-oriented, unstructured treatment. The clinician and the child engage in play activity. As the child says something, the clinician expands it into a different syntactic form than the one the child produced or presumably intended. For example, the child may say "Big ball"; the clinician then might recast this into a question by saying "Is this a big ball?" Or, the clinician might recast it into a negation by saying "No, this is not a big ball." Whether this technique is effective has not been established in controlled studies.

Incidental Teaching

This is a technique conducive to teaching language in more naturalistic settings. It also is useful in latter stages of training when the clinician needs to move on to conversational or less structured treatment. **Incidental teaching** is a procedure in which natural communicative situations are used to reinforce a variety of target behaviors (Hart & Risley, 1982). By this time, the clinician will have trained many kinds of language behaviors using the discrete trial procedure, or other more formal procedures. During conversation, productions of any of the previously trained behaviors may be verbally reinforced. But the clinician does not manipulate any special stimuli to evoke them. There is no modeling. As the child produces a plural /s/ in a natural context, the clinician might say "Good, you said *bats*." The conversational speech is only minimally interrupted by such verbal praise. The interaction is as natural as it can be.

Incidental teaching is an excellent procedure for the parents to use at home. The procedure can be used in many natural conversational situations. It allows for spontaneity. Expansion is frequently used in incidental teaching. For example, when the child says "Mom, I want cookie," the mother may say "Do you want *a* cookie?; I will give you *a* cookie; here is *a* cookie. Take *a* cookie." The mother used the article *a* in different contexts to show how it is a part of many forms of sentences. Some clinicians ask the parent to require a response from the child; others do not. Again, it may be more effective to ask the child to imitate one of the correct responses and reinforce the child. For example, the mother, after having expanded, and just before handing the cookie, might ask, "Say I want *a* cookie." The child might imitate the full response which would be immediately reinforced by the presentation of the cookie.

Incidental teaching can be useful in promoting response generalization and maintenance. Using natural opportunities, parents can teach new behaviors or sustain (reinforce) clinically learned behaviors. There is experimental evidence supporting the effectiveness of incidental teaching.

Mand-Model

This is a variation of the incidental teaching method; therefore, it is a more naturalistic teaching method. Treatment is conducted in play-oriented, naturalistic settings. First, the clinician draws the child's attention to a stimulus such as an attractive toy. Next, the clinician **mands** (request, command, demand) a response from the child by asking the child to "tell me what you want" or "tell me what this is." If the child fails to respond, the clinician then models the correct, complete response. The clinician then prompts the child to imitate the modeled response. The clinician finally reinforces the correct response by handing the toy to the child. There is controlled evidence about its effectiveness (Rogers-Warren & Warren, 1980).

The Cloze or Completion

The classic sentence completion method is used to have the child produce target responses. For example, you can show the picture of a man and that of a woman and then say "This is the picture of a man. But this is the picture of a_____." The child is likely to say "Woman." This is similar to partial modeling.

Joint Book Reading

A technique that exploits children's love for stories read to them from books containing large, colorful pictures is called **joint book reading**. In this procedure, the clinician reads the same story repeatedly so that children will memorize most of it. The clinician uses various prosodic features to draw attention to specific language structures. When the children know the story well, the clinician pauses just before specific expressions in the story that serve as language targets. The children then are prompted to complete the sentences, thus encouraging them to use the target structures. In different readings, the clinician pauses at different junctures to sample a variety of cloze expressions from the children.

In joint book reading, the clinician also may ask the children to "read" the book by looking at the pictures (essentially telling the story through picture prompts). There is some evidence that joint book reading is effective (Kirchner, 1991; Whitehurst et al., 1988).

Script Therapy

Scripts refer to knowledge children have about routine events, episodes, and personal experiences. For instance, a child's knowledge about the routines involved in shopping is a script. Scripts in this sense are not written; they are "mental" representations of events and experiences.

In **script therapy**, such knowledge-based representations are used to teach language skills, especially conversational or narrative skills. Script therapy is similar to **joint action routines (interactions)**.

If a child does not have a well established knowledge of events to be used in treatment, the clinician creates it by recreating the event repeatedly in the clinic. For example, if the child does not have a script of eating out in a restaurant, the event is repeatedly created as a role play so that the child acquires the knowledge (the script).

In using the script therapy, the clinician begins by describing the sequence of a selected event verbally (e.g., taking part in a birthday party). The clinician then assigns roles to each of the children and himself or herself (guests, parents, pizza delivery person). Using props, the clinician acts out the event. The clinician then repeats the event with roles reversed. The event may be repeated until the children are fully familiarized with the event and language expressions used. The clinician then begins to pause as the event is acted out for the children in the group to express themselves to carry the event further. Increasingly complex language structures may be introduced gradually. Each child may be given an opportunity to complete the clinician's expressions as he or she pauses at different junctures.

The method appears more useful in group language therapy. More research is needed to establish its efficacy.

A few related procedures are variations of the script therapy or vice versa. For instance, event structures are similar to scripts; they are used just as scripts in language therapy. An **event structure** is a description of a routine event which is acted out to teach various forms of language.

Joint action routines or interactions also use repetitive and routinized activities in language treatment in the manner described under script therapy.

Whole Language Approach

An approach to language intervention based on a theoretical approach to reading and writing is called the **whole language approach**. The approach recommends that language teaching should not be broken down into speaking, reading, and writing; instead, all aspects of literacy including speaking, listening, reading, and writing should be taught simultaneously as an integrated whole. The approach also recommends that language teaching should include academic goals.

There is a great need to evaluate the effects and efficacy of this approach to clinical language teaching. It is not clear whether whole language is more effective than traditional methods of teaching language to children with language disorders. Available clinical evidence suggests that children with limited language skills benefit from a teaching approach that simplifies the target behaviors. Controlled clinical treatment research is needed to demonstrate that the whole language approach is at least as effective as the other well researched approaches in teaching language to children with language disorders.

The message of the whole language approach that language skills are integrated is well taken. Anytime a skill is broken down into components, the components need to be put together and practiced as a whole. That is why, throughout this book, the emphasis has been on moving treatment to complex, integrated, conversational speech level.

RESPONSE REDUCTION PROCEDURES

Clinicians not only need procedures to increase the target behaviors, but also those to decrease undesirable behaviors. Children in language treatment produce incorrect language responses (as the child who says *book* for *books*) and undesirable general behaviors (such as off-seat behaviors or nonattending behaviors). The clinician needs procedures to reduce both the incorrect language behaviors and undesirable general behaviors. There are two major classes of response reduction procedures: direct and indirect.

Direct Response Reduction Procedures

In direct procedures, a contingency is placed on the behavior that needs to be reduced. In the indirect procedures, no specific contingency is placed on the response to be reduced; instead, a desirable behavior is increased by reinforcement so that the undesirable behavior decreases.

Corrective Feedback. When the child omits the target response or produces an incorrect response, clinicians typically give corrective feedback in the form of verbal "No" or "That is not correct." Such corrective feedback is a part of all treatment sessions. The clinician should give the corrective feedback immediately after the wrong response is produced. Also, the clinician should measure the frequency of target behaviors so that if one type of feedback is ineffective, another type may be selected.

Reinforcement Withdrawal. Withdrawing specific reinforcing stimuli or reinforcing state of affairs is an effective strategy to reduce unwanted behaviors. There are two variations of this basic procedure: Response cost and time-out. Both have been extensively researched and shown to be effective.

Response Cost. In this procedure, a reinforcer the child has earned may be withdrawn every time an incorrect response is made. For example, the clinician may take away a token for every wrong response (the child is reinforced with the presentation of a token for every correct response).

Time-out. In this procedure, the clinician terminates a reinforcing state of affairs. The clinician says

"Stop" as soon as a child makes a wrong response and turns his or her face away from the child for a few seconds (5 to 10 seconds). Then the clinician reestablishes eye contact and continues the conversation or treatment trial presentation.

Extinction. In this procedure, the clinician simply stops reinforcing an undesirable behavior. For example, if the child begins to cry during a treatment session, the clinician simply tells the child that "we can get back to work when you stop crying" and turns his or her back to the child and sits motionless. The clinician does not pay any attention to the child as long as he or she is crying. As soon as the crying stops, the clinician promptly turns toward the child, smiles, reinforces verbally or otherwise, and continues the treatment activity.

Indirect Response Reduction Procedures

As noted earlier, in all indirect procedures, no contingency is placed on the behavior to be reduced; instead, a positive reinforcement contingency is placed on a desirable behavior that indirectly reduces the undesirable behavior. There are several such procedures, only two will be described here.

Differential Reinforcement of Other Behavior. In this procedure, the clinician identifies a behavior that will not be reinforced and any one of several desirable behaviors, none specified, will be reinforced. For example, a clinician might tell a boy who keeps reaching for the stimulus materials on the table that he will not get a token as long as he keeps doing it but will receive a token for not doing it. Note that the instruction does not specify the behavior that will earn the token. The clinician then will give a token if the child keeps his hands on the lap; for keeping his hands on the table; for using his hands to hold the stimulus picture; and so forth. A variety of acceptable behaviors will be reinforced. As a result, the undesirable behavior singled out for nonreinforcement will decrease.

Differential Reinforcement of Incompatible Behavior. In this procedure, the clinician selects for reinforcement a desirable behavior that is physically incompatible with the undesirable behavior. For example, a boy who hits the one sitting next to him may be reinforced for drawing; drawing and hitting are incompatible. A child in language treatment who often leaves the chair may be heavily reinforced for sitting; the two are incompatible. Note that in this procedure, too, the undesirable behavior is reduced indirectly by reinforcing another behavior.

PROCEDURAL MODIFICATIONS

No language treatment procedure is effective all the time with all children. The technique that produces a dramatic effect in a given child on one occasion may not work the next time. By keeping accurate records of the child's progress, you modify the procedures that are not producing the desired effects. You should be prepared to modify all aspects of the treatment program. Thus, you should be prepared to change.

Change Reinforcers and Corrective Feedback Methods

Always remember that there are no standard reinforcers or corrective feedback procedures. A reinforcer should increase the target response rate and corrective feedback should decrease it. If these are not happening, change the reinforcer or the corrective feedback.

Gradually Reduce the Amount of Reinforcement

Initially reinforce every correct response. But gradually reduce the amount of reinforcement. You may reinforce every 4th or 6th response (fixed ratio of 4 or 6). If you used primary reinforcers (food), fade them in gradual steps; you always use verbal praise so that eventually only this reinforcer is used on a "thin" schedule (a fixed ratio of 10, perhaps).

Modify or Change the Target Behavior

Sometimes you find out that the initial target behavior is too complex for the child because the child does not even imitate it. In this case, drop to a lower level of response complexity. For instance, if teaching certain morphological features at the phrase level proves to be too difficult, teach them at the word level. If the feature is too difficult at any level, change to another feature. But return to the difficult feature later on.

Change Stimuli

In some cases, target responses do not increase because the stimuli were ambiguous or unattractive, hence ineffective. In such cases, select better pictures, or if possible, use objects.

A creative clinician is the one who is constantly looking for better procedures and modifying established procedures to produce greater effects. Do not hesitate to change something when the response rates do not show improvement. Always think that it is possible to improve the procedures. Analyze failures at the earliest stage; do not continue with ineffective procedures for any length of time. To do all this, you must be doing one thing in all sessions: measuring the rate of target responses. If you do not, you often do not know what effects your procedures have on the client.

CLASS NOTES

Instructor's Views and Critical Comments on Treatment of Language Disorders: Variations and Additional Procedures _____

_____

_____

_____

_____

_____

_____

_____

_____

_____

_____

_____

_____

_____

_____

_____

_____

_____

_____

_____

_____

_____

_____

_____

_____

REFERENCES AND READING ASSIGNMENTS

Hart, B. B., & Risley, T. R. (1982). *How to use incidental teaching for elaborating language.* Lawrence, KS: H & H Enterprises.

Read this book to fully understand the incidental teaching method.

Hegde, M. N. (1993). *Treatment procedures in communicative disorders* (2nd ed.). Austin, TX: PRO-ED.

Read Chapter 5 for a description of the basic procedure of establishing treatment targets.

Kirchner, D. (1991). Reciprocal book reading. A discourse-based intervention strategy for the child with atypical language development. In T. Gallagher (Ed.), *Pragmatics of language: Clinical practice issues* (pp. 307–332). San Diego: Singular Publishing Group.

Read this article to understand the reciprocal book reading method.

Paul, R. (1995). *Language disorders from infancy through adolescence.* St. Louis: Mosby.

Read sections on treatment in Chapters 7 through 10 for various language treatment techniques.

Reed, V. (1994). *An introduction to children with language disorders* (2nd ed.). New York: Macmillan.

Read Chapter 15 on language intervention (Start at "Approaches to Intervention" on p. 452; read the rest of the chapter).

Rogers-Warren, A., & Warren, S. (1980). Mands for verbalization. *Behavior Modification, 4,* 230–245.

Read this article for details on the Mand-Model approach.

Whitehurst, G., Falco, F., Lonigan, C., Fischel, J., DeBryshe, B., Valdez-Menchaea, M., & Caulfield, M. (1988). Accelerating language development through picture book reading. *Developmental Psychology, 24,* 552–558.

Read this article for one approach to teaching language by picture book reading.

Special Assignments From the Instructor:

_____

_____

_____

_____

_____

_____

_____

_____

_____

_____

_____

_____

_____

_____

_____

_____

_____

_____

_____

_____

STUDY QUESTIONS

1. What are the two options available when a given behavior reaches the tentative training criterion at the lowest level of response topography?

   _____

   _____

   _____

   _____

   _____

   _____

2. Define shaping. Describe how you would use it with an example:

   _____

   _____

   _____

   _____

   _____

   _____

3. What is prompting?

   _____

   _____

   _____

   _____

   _____

   _____

4. What is fading? How do you fade a modeled stimulus?

   _____

   _____

   _____

   _____

   _____

   _____

5. Define each of the following terms; point out how they differ from each other; illustrate each with an example: expansion, extension, and recast:

_____

_____

_____

_____

_____

_____

_____

_____

_____

_____

_____

6. Describe incidental teaching:

_____

_____

_____

_____

_____

_____

_____

_____

7. Describe the mand-model method:

_____

_____

_____

_____

_____

8. What is a script? How is it used in script therapy?

_____

_____

_____

_____

_____

_____

_____

_____

9. What is a cloze procedure? How is it used in therapy?

_____

_____

_____

_____

10. Describe the procedure of joint book reading in treating language disorders:

_____

_____

_____

_____

_____

_____

11. What is the whole language approach?

_____

_____

_____

_____

_____

_____

12. Define response cost. Describe its use:

_____

_____

_____

_____

_____

_____

13. Define time-out. Describe its use:?

_____

_____

_____

_____

_____

14. Define extinction. How is it used?

_____

_____

_____

_____

_____

15. What factors in treatment may have to be changed? What kinds of changes would you do?

_____

_____

_____

_____

_____

_____

_____

_____

Language Treatment: Conversational Skills

. . . .

- Pragmatics and Language Intervention

- Treatment of Conversational Skills

- References and Reading Assignments

- Study Questions

. . . .

PRAGMATICS FAND LANGUAGE INTERVENTION

As noted in earlier units, pragmatics is the study of the social use of language. Pragmatic structures or features refer to various language skills exhibited in natural communicative contexts. These skills make up social conversation. The final goal of language intervention is appropriate and sustained use of conversational skills in social situations.

Treatment of language disorders in children will not be complete until the clinician trains conversational skills and then implements a maintenance program to make those skills last. In Unit 13 you will learn about implementing a maintenance program. In this unit, you will learn about teaching selected pragmatic features, especially the conversational skills.

Any language structure, whether it is a word, a phrase, a sentence, or continuous conversational speech, is an appropriate pragmatic target. That is, a word also should be used appropriately in social situations. However, for the most part, clinicians have focused on conversational skills in pragmatic language training. This is because the words and phrases are the building blocks of conversational speech. When pragmatic training moves into this complex level, skills taught at the lower level are necessarily incorporated into the advanced language skills.

Typically, conversational skills are taught in the later stages of intervention. Most children with language disorders initially need to learn a set of words, morphologic features taught in words, phrases, and sentences, and a variety of syntactic structures. Because the kinds of conversational skills described are components of an advanced language skill, the clinician cannot teach them to a child who has very limited language.

Pragmatic language treatment is not a unique approach to language intervention; it is just taking intervention to a more complex skill level. Nor does the pragmatic approach replace other training targets.

Pragmatic skills build upon semantic, morphologic, and syntactic skills.

There are very few treatment efficacy studies on pragmatic language training. The pragmatic view of language has been mostly theoretical. Therefore, many techniques advocated to teach pragmatic features need to be experimentally evaluated for their immediate effects and long-term efficacy.

TREATMENT OF CONVERSATIONAL SKILLS

The following are among the conversational skills emphasized in advanced, pragmatic language training; train them with the procedures described:

Topic initiation. Starting conversation on a new topic. In effect, it is the initiation of conversation. Most children with language disorders are deficient in this skill; hence it is a treatment target.

Teach topic initiation by using the following general procedure; modify as necessary:

- Use a variety of stimuli to suggest a new topic for conversation; novel and interesting objects, pictures, story books, topic cards (for children who can read), toys, and structured play situations (such as a kitchen) may help trigger conversation

- Draw the child's attention to a manipulated object or an unusual stimulus; show the initial picture of a series of pictures that tell a story

- Give a few seconds for the child to initiate conversation about the stimulus presented

- Tell the child to say something if the child does not initiate a topic

- Prompt the child to start conversation or story telling ("the lion is trying to . . .")

- Reinforce the child for saying anything related to the topic on hand

- Accept initially anything the child might say but shape more relevant responses

- Teach the child to use the topic cards to initiate new topics

- Ask the child to think of new topics to talk about

- Prompt new topics

- Withdraw or fade such prompts, cues, cards, pictures, and other special stimuli to make topic initiation more spontaneous

- Train parents to use the techniques that you find effective with the child

Topic maintenance. Continuing to talk on the same topic for socially acceptable or appropriate durations. The duration is variable and dependent upon the individual conversational episode. This is a skill to be taught because most children with language disorders do not maintain a topic of conversation for extended durations.

Teach topic maintenance by using the following general procedure; modify as necessary:

- Offer various topics for conversation initially and ask the child to select one; later on, prompt the child to suggest a topic; finally, fade prompting to let the child spontaneously suggest a topic

- Select initially a brief duration for which you want the child to talk on a single topic; or set a target number of words to be produced on a topic

- Shape increased duration of conversation or increased number of words

- Use such devices as *tell me more, say more, what about that, what happened next, who said what, who did what, where did it happen, how did it happen* and so forth to stimulate more speech on the same topic

- Reinforce the child for talking continuously on the same topic

- Say "Stop" when the child abruptly switches the topic; ask more details or ask questions about the same topic to encourage the child to return to the topic

- Complete training on multiple topics and then probe with untrained topics to see if the skills have generalized

- Introduce new topics for training if the skills have not generalized

- Train parents to teach topic maintenance at home

Turn Taking. Playing the role of talker and listener in an alternating manner. This is a conversational skill to be taught because most children with language disorders do not take turns appropriately.

Teach turn taking by using the following general procedure; modify as necessary:

- Baserate the correct and incorrect instances of turn taking

- Use a verbal ("Your turn") or nonverbal signal (a hand gesture to suggest *you speak*) for the child to talk

- Give a signal that says do not interrupt and do not talk (e.g., finger on your lips)

- Use a real or a toy microphone as a discriminative stimulus to teach the role of a speaker; exchange it with the child; teach the child to speak only when holding the microphone and to listen when the other person is holding it

- Reinforce the child for correct turn taking (talking only when signaled or while holding the microphone)

- Do not violate the rule you impose on the child (e.g., talk only when you hold the microphone)

- Teach the child to say "it is your turn" or signal it in some way

- Reinforce the child for letting you talk ("thank you for letting me take my turn")

- Teach turn taking until the child meets a performance criterion (e.g., no errors of turn taking in two consecutive conversational exchanges)

- Fade the signals and the special discriminative stimuli used to prompt the child

- Probe without signals or special discriminative stimuli

Train until a probe criterion is met (at least 90% accuracy in turn taking while not receiving reinforcers)

Conversational Repair Strategies. Skills in overcoming breakdowns in conversational communication. Includes such skills as requesting for clarification when a speaker's statements are not clear and varying one's expressions when a listener does not understand. This is a pragmatic skill to be taught because children with language disorders do not know how to get clarifications from speakers and how to vary their own productions when their listeners ask for clarifications.

Teach the following two conversational repair strategies by using the procedures suggested; modify as necessary.

Teach the child to **request clarifications** from a speaker:

- Make ambiguous statements (e.g., "give me the car" when there are several toy cars displayed)

- Wait for the child to request clarification

- If the child does not request clarification and responds anyway (such as picking one of the cars), say "No"

- Wait for the child to request clarification

- If the child does not request clarification, model a response for the child (e.g., "When you are not sure, I want you to ask me 'what do you mean?' OK?")

- Make another ambiguous statement

- Immediately model the request for clarification for the child

- Reinforce the child for imitating the request for clarification (e.g., "What do you mean?")

- Make another ambiguous statement

- Prompt (not model) a request for clarification (e.g., "What do you ask me?")

- Reinforce the child for asking for clarification (e.g., "What do you mean?")

- Introduce varied ambiguous statements

- Fade modeling and prompting

- Train parents in teaching the child to request for clarification

Teach the child to **vary the expressions** when requested by a listener; you play the role of a listener who does not fully understand the expressions of the child:

- Ask the child to repeat

- Ask the child "What do you mean?"

- Tell the child "I do not understand"

- Negate a child's utterance so the child will clarify by assertion ("You did not go on the roller coaster 20 times did you?"; the child might say "No, I went on it two times")

- Model the clarified statement by modifying what the child said ("You mean you went on the roller coaster two times, right?")

- Rephrase the child's utterance into a question and say it with a rising intonation ("You went on the roller coaster 20 times?")

- Model different ways of saying the same thing

- Ask the child to say it differently; reinforce varied phrases or sentences

- Periodically stop responding to prompt the child to rephrase (e.g., rephrasing an ambiguous request)

- Train parents to prompt the child to vary expressions and to reinforce the child for compliance

Narrative Skills. Story telling, narrating personal experiences. Logical consistency, correct temporal sequence, movement from beginning to the end, and so forth are the specific skills involved in narrative skills. These skills need to be taught because children with language disorders often cannot narrate experiences and events.

Teach narrative skills by using the following general procedure; modify as necessary:

- Tell the child a brief story and ask the child to retell it

- Take note of the missing elements or wrong temporal sequences as the child retells

- Tell the same story again to the child

- Ask the child to retell the story with the help of pictures that prompt the story events

- Stop the child when the sequence is wrong

- Prompt the correct sequence of events

- Stop the child when an important element is missed in the sequence

- Prompt the child to include the missing element

- Reinforce the child for appropriate narrative skills

- Use different and progressively longer stories as the child's narrative skills improve

- Fade the use of pictures

- Shift training to describing personal events

- Stop and prompt the child as appropriate and necessary

- Fade stopping and prompting

- Probe with new stories and experiences

- Pause at important junctures as you tell a story so the child can supply narrative portions

- Use the **script therapy** described in Unit 11 to give children experience in establishing scripts (schemes of events), also described in the same unit

Eye contact. Maintaining eye contact with the listener during conversation. A conversational skill to be taught because children with language disorders often do not maintain eye contact; may be cultural as well.

If the child's lack of eye contact is cultural, discuss this with parents; teach it if they agree to the target. Teach eye contact by using the following general procedure; modify as necessary:

- Instruct the child about eye contact

- Model eye contact during conversation

- Prompt the child to maintain eye contact

- Use such standard phrases as "Look at me" as soon as the child begins to talk

- Immediately reinforce the child for making eye contact

- Shape longer durations of eye contact

Integrated Conversational Skill. Appropriate use of individually taught conversational skills in integrated conversational episodes. When such specific skills as topic maintenance and turn taking are taught, the clinician needs to shift training to conversational episodes that incorporate all previously taught skills.

- Ask the child to suggest a topic for conversation

- Suggest a conversational topic if the child fails to initiate a topic

- Use topic cards and picture books only when more natural means are not effective in initiating a topic of conversation

- Reinforce the child for maintaining eye contact during conversation

- Ask questions about the topic, request the child to say more, and prompt subtopics to keep the child on the same topic for an extended period of time

- Reinforce the child for continuing to talk on a specific topic

- Remind and reinforce the child to take turns

- Say "No" or "Stop" when the child interrupts your speech (inappropriate turn taking)

- Make ambiguous statements to prompt the child to ask questions or request clarifications

- Reinforce the child's questions or requests

- Ask the child for elaborations or clarifications

- Reinforce the child for making elaborations and providing clarifications

- Ask the child to narrate a personal experience

- Prompt the child to use the skills previously taught regarding narration

- Reinforce the child for appropriate narrative skills

- Integrate other pragmatic skills taught

Conversational Skills in Naturalistic Settings. The final goal of language intervention. Informal training of conversational skills in extraclinical situations and training significant others in maintaining conversational skills in those situations are the two most important components of this level of intervention.

- Use the method described under **Integrated Conversational Skill**

- Use those methods as you shift training from the clinical setting to nonclinical settings

- Engage the child in conversation outside the clinic

- Engage the child in conversation in such places as the library, cafeteria, classroom, and other settings

- Take the child for a walk on the campus or around the clinic and engage the child in conversation

- Train parents to conduct similar conversational training sessions at home

- Reinforce the child for using all the specific conversational skills

- Train parents in reinforcement and response maintenance procedures

Instructor's Views and Critical Comments on Treatment of Conversational Skills

REFERENCES AND READING ASSIGNMENTS

Duchan, J. F., Hewitt, L. E., & Sonnenmeir, R. M. (Eds.). (1994). *Pragmatics: From theory to practice.* Englewood Cliffs, NJ: Prentice-Hall.

Read the various chapters in this book on pragmatic language intervention techniques.

Gallagher, T. (Ed.). (1991). *Pragmatics of language: Clinical practice issues.* San Diego: Singular Publishing Group.

Read the various chapters in this book on pragmatic language intervention techniques.

Hegde, M. N. (1996). *A pocketguide to treatment procedures in speech-language pathology.* San Diego: Singular Publishing Group.

Read the alphabetized entry on language disorders in children.

Nelson, N. W. (1993). *Childhood language disorders in context.* New York: Macmillan.

Read sections of Chapter 8 on pragmatic features.

Paul, R. (1995). *Language disorders from infancy through adolescence.* St. Louis: Mosby.

Read sections of Chapters 10 and 13 on pragmatics.

Special Assignments From the Instructor:

_____

_____

_____

_____

_____

_____

_____

_____

_____

_____

_____

_____

_____

_____

_____

_____

_____

_____

_____

_____

_____

_____

STUDY QUESTIONS

1. Define the following terms:

   Pragmatics _____

   _____

   _____

   Topic initiation _____

   _____

   _____

   Topic maintenance _____

   _____

   _____

   Turn taking _____

   _____

   _____

   Narrative skills _____

   _____

   _____

   Conversational repair strategies _____

   _____

   _____

   _____

2. Describe the steps you would take in teaching a child to initiate conversation on a given topic:

   _____

   _____

   _____

   _____

   _____

   _____

3. Describe the procedures for teaching topic maintenance:

_____

_____

_____

_____

_____

_____

_____

_____

4. Describe the procedures for teaching conversational turn taking:

_____

_____

_____

_____

_____

5. Describe the procedures for teaching a child to request for clarification:

_____

_____

_____

_____

_____

_____

_____

6. Describe the procedures for teaching a child to vary his or her own utterances in response to request for clarification:

_____

_____

_____

_____

_____

_____

_____

_____

7. Describe how you would integrate different conversational skills:

_____

_____

_____

_____

_____

_____

_____

_____

8. Describe the procedures for teaching a child to use conversational skills in natural settings:

_____

_____

_____

_____

_____

_____

_____

_____

Maintenance Strategies

....

- Definition of a Clinical Problem

- Strategies for Response Maintenance

- References and Reading Assignments

- Study Questions

....

In this final unit, you will learn how to make the newly taught language skills last in the client's natural environment.

DEFINITION OF A CLINICAL PROBLEM

With the help of the clinician, children often learn new language skills in a structured, clinical situation. It is in the clinician's office, a special classroom setting, or a special treatment room that the skills are established. Unfortunately, the problem that still remains is that the newly established behaviors may not be produced in the child's home, school, the playground, and other naturalistic settings. Sometimes, the new behaviors that are initially produced in the naturalistic settings may be lost over time; they may not be maintained.

The lack of newly learned behaviors in the naturalistic settings has been traditionally labeled a **problem of generalization**. That is, the behaviors learned in one setting do not generalize to other settings. The problem also has been labeled as one of **carryover** (the behaviors are not "carried-over.")

Generalization is a learning phenomenon. A response learned in the context of one stimulus may be produced in the context of other, similar stimuli. Such productions are called **stimulus generalization**. The behavior learned in one physical setting may be exhibited in other, similar settings though there was no conditioning in those other settings. This is called **setting generalization**.

A new response similar to the one just taught also may be exhibited. This is called **response generalization**. If one person teaches a response and the response is made in the presence of another person, we have a variety of stimulus generalization. Therefore, it appears that generalization is what is lacking when children fail to produce the clinically established behaviors in their home and other settings. Therefore, clinicians asserted that the final goal of clinical intervention is generalization.

UNIT NOTES

CLASS NOTES

When you examine the concept of generalization carefully, however, you will find that generalization should not be the final goal of clinical intervention (Hegde, 1993). Defined according to laboratory data, **generalization is a declining rate of response when the stimuli are changed and the responses are not reinforced**. No generalized response lasts forever unless it is reinforced; technically, generalized responses are not reinforced. Left to run its natural course, a generalized response is extinguished. If a response is reinforced, then it is teaching, conditioning, learning, but not generalization.

Therefore, the final target of treatment is maintenance of clinically established behaviors in naturalistic settings. Language behaviors taught in the clinic should be exhibited in typical conversations produced in a variety of everyday situations. The behaviors must be maintained over time, not just generalized. To maintain those responses, we need to reinforce them. This reinforcement must come not from the clinician who is not there (in the naturalistic settings), but from the people who live with the client (family members) or those who are in everyday contact with the client (friends, teachers, colleagues).

When it does occur, generalization can be helpful in promoting maintenance. For example, when a behavior taught in the clinic is produced in a naturalistic setting perhaps because of stimulus similarity, the parents then can reinforce it and thus make the behavior last. However, asking parents and others to reinforce a generalized response is not a strategy to promote generalization; it is a strategy to extend treatment to natural settings.

Promoting generalization is desirable only because generalization can serve as a foundation for maintenance strategies. We know of many variables that initially produce generalization. These variables can be incorporated into treatment with the hope that maintenance strategies can then be implemented more easily. This seems to be about the only use we have of the concept of generalization in treatment.

Reinforcement of behaviors in homes by family members is the same as reinforcement of behaviors in clinics by clinicians. There is no reason to call one the strategy to promote generalization and the other treatment. Both are treatment and only treatment can make behaviors last.

STRATEGIES FOR RESPONSE MAINTENANCE

The clinician can implement a variety of procedures to make the response last in naturalistic settings. This is not to say the problem of response maintenance has been solved; much research is needed before this important clinical problem can be solved. Meanwhile, research has shown the usefulness of many procedures that the clinician can use. Most of these procedures require that you extend treatment to naturalistic settings. That is why **maintenance strategy** may be defined as an extension of treatment to naturalistic settings.

To promote maintenance, existing interactional patterns of the child and his or her family members and significant others should be changed. The family members and others should now act and react differently. They should set the stage for the child to exhibit the newly learned language skills. They then should support it by social approval and natural consequences. They should stop supporting the child's old and ineffective ways of communication.

The basic idea behind the maintenance strategy is that treatment settings and natural settings are different. The clinical setting will have created new contexts, stimuli, and settings for new language skills and new, supportive consequences for using those skills. The natural setting, on the other hand, may continue with old stimuli and context that supported inappropriate or deficient language skills. The people in the natural setting may not know how to evoke and strengthen the newly established language skills. Therefore, the skills may not be maintained beyond the clinical setting.

The main task of the clinician in implementing a maintenance strategy is to diminish the differences between the clinical and natural settings and to train significant others to sustain and support the new skills.

To promote initial generalization and eventual maintenance of target skills, the clinician should:

- Think of maintenance from the very beginning of treatment, not after the establishment of target behaviors.

- Select client-specific responses that are useful. Teach behaviors that can be expected to be produced at home and in classrooms.

- Teach each target behavior with multiple exemplars (several contexts in which the preposition *on* is taught, for example).

- Select stimuli (used in evoking the target responses) from the child's natural environment. For instance, the child's toy car is a better stimulus for the word *car* than a picture selected from the clinician's cupboard.

- Select verbal antecedents that are common (ask common questions to evoke target behaviors, for example).

- Bring teachers and family members to the treatment sessions. Have the child produce the target behaviors in the presence of a different audience.

- Move treatment to more natural and less structured situations as soon as possible. Informally monitor the child's production of target behaviors in the playground, school cafeteria, classroom, hallway, shopping center, restaurant, and the child's home.

- Reduce the initial continuous reinforcement. In gradual steps, shift reinforcement to an intermittent schedule; stretch the schedule gradually.

- Use social and natural consequences of communication as reinforcers, especially in the latter stages of treatment. Use verbal reinforcers even when primary reinforcers are used.

- Delay reinforcement in the final stages of treatment. Increase the duration of delay in gradual steps.

- Reinforce complex verbal responses in the conversational mode in the latter stages of treatment.

- Train the significant others in contingency management; train parents, siblings, friends, teachers, and others to reinforce the production of correct language behaviors.

- Teach self-control or self-monitoring procedures. Teach the child to chart his or her correct and incorrect responses. Teach the child to recognize his or her mistakes and self-correct.

- Teach the child to prompt the ignoring parents or teachers to reinforce his or her correct production by drawing attention to it (e.g., *"Mom, I said two cups, not two cup"* followed by attention and praise from the mother).

- Provide an adequate amount of treatment to promote maintenance because often it is insufficient treatment that causes lack of maintenance.

- Follow-up the child periodically. Reassess the target behaviors during the follow-up. Offer booster treatment if the target skills are not maintained.

Maintenance can be achieved only by implementing a variety of procedures. Varying training stimuli, training settings, target behaviors, audience for those behaviors, and reinforcement schedule all follow the same theme: do not teach a limited set of responses under limited stimulus conditions. Eventually, significant others should act in such a way as to support and maintain the skills in the child's environment. Therefore, parental (or family) involvement in treatment is a key factor. In the school setting, the clinician should work closely with teachers, peers, and family members. Eventually, they have to maintain the language skills until the skills come under the influence of many natural contingencies. That is why it is important to teach them how to recognize and reinforce appropriate language behaviors, not just the ones the clinician has taught the child. The other key factor is self-monitoring. Even the parents will not be available all the time to monitor the correct behavior productions. The client is his or her only constant companion. Therefore, it is the client who must monitor the behaviors all the time.

Instructor's Views and Critical Comments on Treatment of Language Disorders: Generalization and Maintenance

REFERENCES AND READING ASSIGNMENTS

Hegde, M. N. (1993). *Treatment procedures in communicative disorders* (2nd ed.). Austin, TX: PRO-ED.

Read Chapter 7 on discrimination, generalization, and maintenance.

Reed, V. (1994). *An introduction to children with language disorders* (2nd ed.). New York: Macmillan.

Read the section entitled "Generalization" in Chapter 15 (pp. 450–451).

Special Assignments From the Instructor:

_____

_____

_____

_____

_____

_____

_____

_____

_____

_____

_____

_____

_____

_____

_____

_____

_____

_____

_____

_____

STUDY QUESTIONS

1. What is a major problem faced by speech-language clinicians in the treatment of language disorders?

   _____

   _____

   _____

   _____

2. How has this problem been traditionally labeled?

   _____

   _____

   _____

3. What is stimulus generalization?

   _____

   _____

   _____

4. What is setting generalization?

   _____

   _____

   _____

5. How was generalization defined in this Unit?

   _____

   _____

   _____

6. What does it mean to say that generalization must be our final clinical target?:

   _____

   _____

   _____

   _____

7. According to this Unit, what is the suggested final clinical target?

_____

_____

_____

_____

8. Why is generalization not a final target of clinical intervention?

_____

_____

_____

_____

9. What kinds of target responses should you select?

_____

_____

_____

_____

10. What kinds of stimuli should you select?

_____

_____

_____

_____

11. What is meant by multiple exemplars?

_____

_____

_____

_____

12. What kinds of verbal antecedents do you select?

_____

_____

_____

_____

13. Why should you bring other persons to treatment sessions?

_____

_____

_____

_____

14. Do you continue treatment in your office until the child is dismissed?

_____

_____

_____

_____

15. If your answer to #14 is *No*, what do you do?

_____

_____

_____

_____

16. Describe the reinforcement schedules you would use in the beginning and later stages of treatment:

_____

_____

_____

_____

17. What kinds of reinforcers do you use in the latter stages of treatment? In all stages?

_____

_____

_____

_____

18. Why should you train the "significant others" in contingency management?

_____

_____

_____

_____

19. What is meant by training the significant others?

_____

_____

_____

_____

20. What is a self-monitoring skill you would teach a client?

_____

_____

_____

_____

21. What do you do when a response does generalize?

_____

_____

_____

_____

22. In the latter stages of treatment, what kinds of verbal responses are reinforced?

_____

_____

_____

_____

23. Do you always reinforce immediately? Explain your answer:

_____

_____

_____

_____

24. What is the purpose of follow-up?

_____

_____

_____

_____

25. What is booster treatment?

_____

_____

_____

_____